CONTENTS

Chapter 1 Diet and Health

Chapter 2 Ethical Eating

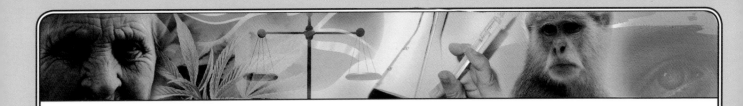

OTHER TITLES IN THE ISSUES SERIES

For more on these titles, visit: www.independence.co.uk

A note on critical evaluation

Because the information reprinted here is from a number of different sources, readers should bear in mind the origin of the text and whether the source is likely to have a particular bias when presenting information (just as they would if undertaking their own research). It is hoped that, as you read about the many aspects of the issues explored in this book, you will critically evaluate the information presented. It is important that you decide whether you are being presented with facts or opinions. Does the writer give a biased or an unbiased report? If an opinion is being expressed, do you agree with the writer?

Nutrition and Diet offers a useful starting point for those who need convenient access to information about the many issues involved. However, it is only a starting point. Following each article is a URL to the relevant organisation's website, which you may wish to visit for further information.

Nutrition and Diet

ISSUES

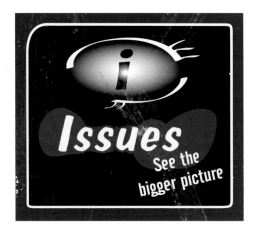

Volume 205

Series Editor

Lisa Firth

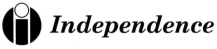
Independence

Educational Publishers

Cambridge

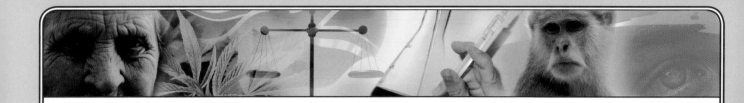

First published by Independence

The Studio, High Green

Great Shelford

Cambridge CB22 5EG

England

© Independence 2011

British Library Cataloguing in Publication Data

Nutrition and diet. -- (Issues ; v. 205)

1. Diet--Great Britain. 2. Food habits--Great Britain.

3. Nutrition--Great Britain. 4. Food industry and trade--

Safety regulations--Great Britain. 5. Food contamination.

I. Series II. Firth, Lisa.

613.2-dc22

ISBN-13: 978 1 86168 577 3

Printed in Great Britain

MWL Print Group Ltd

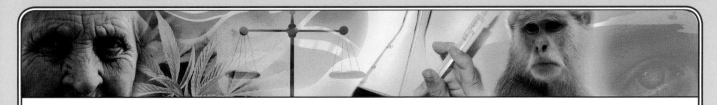

The nation's diet

National Diet and Nutrition Survey *published.*

Results from the first year of the new *National Diet and Nutrition Survey (NDNS)* suggest that the UK population is eating less saturated fat, less trans fat and less added sugar than it was ten years ago.

Saturated fat intakes in adults have dropped slightly to 12.8% of food energy, compared with 13.3% in 2000/01, and men and children are eating less added sugar.

The population's trans fat intakes have also fallen slightly and are now at 0.8% of food energy, which is well within recommended levels. And, on average, adults are eating 4.4 portions of fruit and vegetables a day with over a third of men and women now meeting the 'five-a-day' guideline.

However, despite these encouraging indications, intakes of saturated fat are still above the recommended level of 11% of food energy intake, and at 12.5%, population intakes of added sugars still exceed the recommended 11%.

The research shows that the overall picture of the diet and nutrition of the UK population is broadly similar to previous surveys in the *NDNS* series carried out between 1992 and 2001, although there are suggestions of positive changes. Importantly though, the findings do not identify any new or emerging nutritional problems in the general population.

Other findings include:

⇨ People are still not eating enough fibre, which is essential for healthy digestion. Current average intakes are 14g per day for adults, some way below the recommended 18g.

⇨ Consumption of oily fish, which is the main source of beneficial omega 3 fatty acids, remains low. Both adults and children are eating well below the recommendation of one portion per week.

⇨ Iron intakes among girls aged 11 to 18 years and women are still low in many cases – which can lead to iron deficiency and anaemia. However, overall, vitamin and mineral intakes among the population are slightly improved.

Gill Fine, Director of Consumer Choice and Dietary Health at the FSA, said: 'The results from the first year of our new *NDNS* rolling programme provide us with an interesting snapshot of the nation's diet, and will allow us to track emerging trends over future years. The evidence from this and from further surveys will help us and other government departments formulate policy to address the issues that have been raised.

'It's good news that the survey suggests around a third of the population is eating five portions of fruit and veg each day and it's encouraging to see that these initial findings suggest slightly lower intakes of saturated fat and added sugars than in previous surveys. However, there is obviously a way to go before we are meeting all the Government's dietary recommendations.

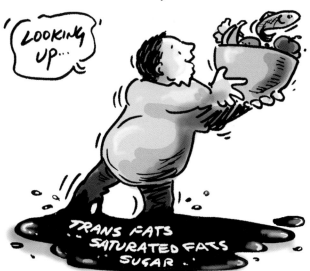

'Good nutrition is important for health and poor diet accounts for a large percentage of premature deaths. We now need to build on the indications of positive change we have observed in this survey. By continuing our programme of campaign work and encouraging product reformulation in key areas such as saturated fat, we will hopefully observe further improvements over the next few years of the programme.'

9 February 2010

⇨ The above information is reprinted with kind permission from the Food Standards Agency. Visit www.food.gov.uk for more information.

FOOD STANDARDS AGENCY

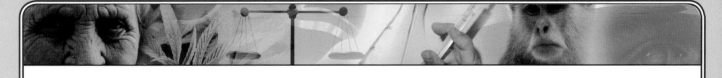

A balanced diet

Despite what you see in some diet books and TV programmes, healthy eating can be really straightforward.

A diet based on starchy foods such as rice and pasta, with plenty of fruit and vegetables, some protein-rich foods such as meat, fish and lentils, and some milk and dairy foods (and not too much fat, salt or sugar) will give you all the nutrients that you need.

When it comes to a healthy diet, balance is the key to getting it right. This means eating a wide variety of foods in the right proportions.

But achieving that balance in modern life can be tricky. After a long day, it can be tempting to grab the first ready meal on the supermarket shelf, which is OK occasionally. But the nutritional labels on these foods show that many ready meals contain high levels of fat, added sugar and salt. If you eat ready meals too often, they'll upset the balance in your diet.

Food groups

The eatwell plate

⇨ To help you get the right balance of the five main food groups, take a look at the Food Standards Agency's eatwell plate below.

⇨ To maintain a healthy diet, the eatwell plate shows you how much of what you eat should come from each food group.

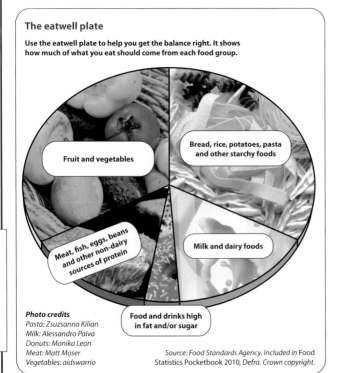

The eatwell plate

Use the eatwell plate to help you get the balance right. It shows how much of what you eat should come from each food group.

Fruit and vegetables

Bread, rice, potatoes, pasta and other starchy foods

Meat, fish, eggs, beans and other non-dairy sources of protein

Milk and dairy foods

Food and drinks high in fat and/or sugar

Photo credits
Pasta: Zsuzsanna Kilian
Milk: Alessandro Paiva
Donuts: Monika Leon
Meat: Matt Moser
Vegetables: aidswarrio

Source: Food Standards Agency. Included in Food Statistics Pocketbook 2010, Defra. Crown copyright.

All the food we eat can be divided into five groups. In a healthy diet you eat the right balance of these groups.

They are:

⇨ Fruit and vegetables.

⇨ Starchy foods, such as rice, pasta, bread and potatoes. Choose wholegrain varieties whenever you can.

⇨ Meat, fish, eggs and beans.

⇨ Milk and dairy foods.

⇨ Foods containing fat and sugar.

Most people in the UK eat too much fat, sugar and salt, and not enough fruit, vegetables and fibre.

1. Fruit and vegetables

Fruit and vegetables are a vital source of vitamins and minerals. It's advised that we eat five portions of a variety of fruit and vegetables a day.

> ## *Most people in the UK eat too much fat, sugar and salt, and not enough fruit, vegetables and fibre*

There's evidence that people who eat at least five portions a day are at lower risk of heart disease, stroke and some cancers.

What's more, eating five portions is not as hard as it might sound. Just one apple, banana, pear or similar-sized fruit is one portion. A slice of pineapple or melon is one portion. Three heaped tablespoons of vegetables is another portion.

Having a sliced banana with your morning cereal is a quick way to get one portion. Swap your mid-morning biscuit for a tangerine, and add a side salad to your lunch. Add a portion of vegetables to dinner, and snack on dried fruit in the evening to reach your five a day.

2. Starchy foods

Starchy foods such as bread, cereals, potatoes, pasta, maize and cornbread are an important part of a healthy diet. They are a good source of energy and the main source of a range of nutrients in our diet. Starchy foods are fuel for your body.

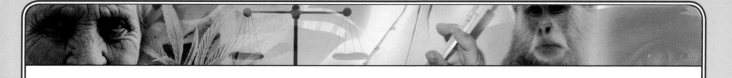

Starchy foods should make up around one-third of everything we eat. This means we should base our meals on these foods.

Try and choose wholegrain or wholemeal varieties, such as brown rice, wholewheat pasta and brown wholemeal bread. They contain more fibre (often referred to as 'roughage'), and usually more vitamins and minerals than white varieties.

Fibre is also found in beans, lentils and peas.

3. Meat, fish, eggs and beans

These foods are all good sources of protein, which is essential for growth and repair of the body. They are also good sources of a range of vitamins and minerals.

Around 15% of the calories that we eat each day should come from protein.

Meat is a good source of protein, vitamins and minerals such as iron, zinc and B vitamins. It is also one of the main sources of vitamin B12. Try to eat lean cuts of meat and skinless poultry whenever possible to cut down on fat. Always cook meat thoroughly.

Fish is another important source of protein, and contains many vitamins and minerals. Oily fish is particularly rich in omega-3 fatty acids.

Aim for at least two portions of fish a week, including one portion of oily fish. You can choose from fresh, frozen or canned, but canned and smoked fish can be high in salt. For more detailed information on the health benefits of eating fish and shellfish and on how much to eat, see Eatwell's fish and shellfish pages (www.eatwell. gov.uk/healthydiet/nutritionessentials/fishandshellfish).

Eggs and pulses (including beans, nuts and seeds) are also great sources of protein. Nuts are high in fibre and a good alternative to snacks high in saturated fat, but they do still contain high levels of fat, so eat them in moderation.

4. Milk and dairy foods

Milk and dairy foods such as cheese and yoghurt are good sources of protein. They also contain calcium, which helps to keep your bones healthy.

But some dairy products are high in saturated fat. Eating too much saturated fat can raise blood cholesterol levels and increase the risk of heart disease. To enjoy the health benefits of dairy without eating too much fat, use semi-skimmed milk, skimmed milk or 1% fat milks, lower-fat hard cheeses or cottage cheese, and lower-fat yoghurt.

5. Fat and sugar

Most people in the UK eat too much fat and too much sugar.

Fats and sugar are both good sources of energy for the body. But when we eat too much of them we consume more energy than we burn, and this can mean that we put on weight. This can lead to obesity, which increases our risk of type 2 diabetes, heart disease and certain cancers.

But did you know that there are different types of fat?

Saturated fat is found in foods such as pies, meat products, sausages, cheese, butter, cakes and biscuits. It can raise your blood cholesterol level and increase your risk of heart disease. Most people in the UK eat too much saturated fat, which puts us at risk of health problems.

Unsaturated fats, on the other hand, can help to lower cholesterol and provide us with the essential fatty acids needed to help us stay healthy. Oily fish, nuts and seeds, avocados, olive oils and vegetable oils are sources of unsaturated fat.

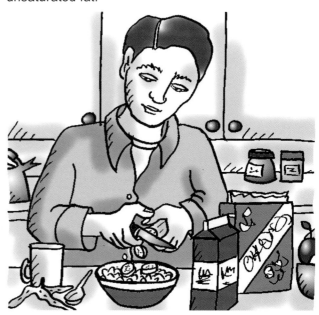

Sugar occurs naturally in foods such as fruit and milk, but we don't need to cut down on these types of sugar. Sugar is also added to lots of foods and drinks such as fizzy drinks, cakes, biscuits, chocolate, pastries, ice cream and jam. It's also contained in some ready-made savoury foods such as pasta sauces and baked beans.

Most of us need to cut down on the foods with added sugar. Instead of a fizzy drink, for example, have a 100% fruit juice diluted with water. Make a pasta sauce yourself instead of buying a ready-made one. Have dried fruit for a snack instead of a chocolate bar.

There are many ways you can cut down on the amount of fat and sugar in your diet.

19 February 2010

⇨ Reproduced by kind permission of the Department of Health.

NHS CHOICES

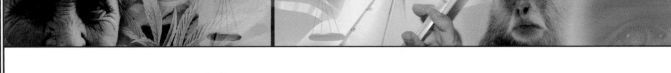

Diet and nutrition

Eating sensibly is an important step towards good health. The more balanced and nutritious the diet, the healthier the person can expect to be.

A healthy balanced diet means eating a wide variety of foods from the four main food groups. These include:

⇨ plenty of fruit and vegetables;

⇨ plenty of starchy foods such as wholegrain bread, pasta and rice;

⇨ some protein-rich foods such as meat, fish, eggs and lentils;

⇨ some dairy foods (ideally reduced fat);

⇨ diets should also be low in fat (especially saturated fats), salt and sugar.

However, a significant proportion of the population (particularly those on low incomes) do not currently meet dietary recommendations. As a result, an estimated one-third of cancers can be attributed to poor diet and nutrition.

The most important aspects of a healthy diet are:

⇨ Choosing foods in the right proportions from the four main food groups.

⇨ Eating a wide variety of different foods and the right amount to maintain a healthy weight.

⇨ Limiting the consumption of other foodstuffs in addition to main meals – especially those which provide a lot of calories, e.g. alcohol and saturated fats, or have little nutritional benefit, such as salt – which can cause health problems in the long term.

The main food groups

There are four main food groups and each one contains nutrients that are essential for growth, energy and body maintenance. The eatwell plate on page 2 is an illustration of what an overall healthy balanced diet should look like. It shows the types and proportion of foods which make up a well-balanced diet. About a third of our food should be starchy foods like bread, potatoes, rice and pasta, and a third should be fruit and vegetables. A healthy diet also includes moderate amounts of meat, fish and alternatives, and moderate amounts of milk and dairy foods – ideally choosing lower fat versions wherever possible. High fat foods and food and drinks containing sugar constitute another

food group but are not essential to a balanced diet and therefore should be eaten sparingly.

Eating at least five portions of fruit and vegetables a day can reduce the risk of heart disease, stroke and some cancers by up to 20%.

Vitamins and minerals

Most people are able to meet their nutritional needs by eating a balanced, varied diet which includes plenty of fruit and vegetables. Therefore they do not need to take dietary supplements. Key exceptions are:

⇨ Women who are, or might become, pregnant are advised to take supplements of folic acid before conception and until the 12th week of pregnancy to help prevent neural tube defects.

RIGHT...I GOT OFF THE COUCH AND OPENED THE REFRIGERATOR DOOR– THAT'S ENOUGH EXERCISE FOR ANYONE!

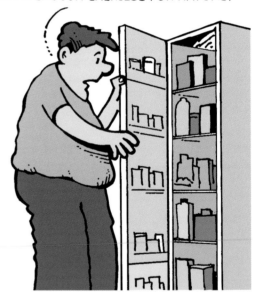

⇨ Pregnant and breastfeeding mothers, young children, people over the age of 65 and those at risk of inadequate sunshine exposure are routinely advised to take supplements of vitamin D as they are more prone to deficiency.

⇨ Women (particularly during pregnancy) or children with iron deficiency anaemia, which has not been found to improve by dietary changes, may be prescribed iron supplements. More information on vitamins and minerals is provided at www.eatwell. gov.uk

PHARMACYHEALTHLINK

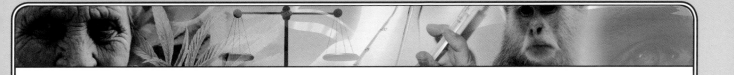

Other foodstuffs

It is important to encourage people to think about other food or drink they have on a regular basis that may affect their health. For example, alcohol, sugary soft drinks and high-salt foods.

Salt

A reduction in the average intake of the overall population from 9g to 6g per day would result in an estimated reduced incidence of coronary heart disease by 6%, stroke by 15% and hypertension by 17%. As most salt in the diet (around 75%) is already in the food we buy, advise people to check the label on food products and choose those lowest in salt. Salt is often listed on food labels as sodium. High salt content is 1.5g or more per 100g (=0.6g sodium or more per 100g).

Alcohol

Alcohol can provide a very high number of calories per day depending on what people drink and how much. Lager, beer and stout have the highest amount of calories per drink and can range from 170 to 400 calories per pint. Therefore it is possible to exceed the maximum daily calorie intake (2000 a day for women and 2500 a day for men) with alcohol alone. In this instance, the person is also likely to be drinking in excess of the recommended daily amount of alcohol, which is two to three units a day for women and three to four units a day for men.

Soft drinks

Fizzy drinks, squashes, 'sports' and 'high juice' drinks all count as soft drinks. They are typically high in sugar (except 'diet' versions) and therefore calories and have very little nutritional value in contrast to 100% fruit juice and smoothies. They also tend to be acidic which can cause tooth decay and enamel erosion if consumed regularly between meals. Healthier alternatives are water, milk and fruit juices (ideally consumed with a meal). Fruit juices should be consumed at meal times because of their high sugar content.

⇨ Information from PharmacyHealthLink. Visit www. phlink.org.uk for more.

© PharmacyHealthLink

Food poisoning

Information from the Food Ethics Council.

According to the Cabinet Office report *Food Matters*, food is as safe as it has ever been. Nevertheless, it is estimated that there are still around 765,000 cases of food poisoning each year in England and Wales and although the rate is declining, deaths due to Listeria are increasing.

Microbiological contamination of meat supply chains is a continuing challenge, as is the threat of diseases transferring to humans from animals and poultry (including avian influenza).

Most food poisoning is due to microbiological contamination (such as chicken contaminated with Campylobacter bacteria) rather than chemical contamination (like harmful dyes or environmental contaminants). But reducing microbiological contamination of certain foods, particularly poultry, remains a real challenge.

Ethical argument

Intensive poultry farming and animal rearing makes it difficult to trace food back to its source, distances food manufacturers from the environmental and social impacts of their products, and puts consumer health and safety at risk.

By treating meat as a commodity and sourcing bulk processed foods through international supply chains, a mixture of meat or chicken from around the world can end up in one burger or chicken nugget. This can make it virtually impossible to identify the source of a food poisoning outbreak.

To ensure a reduction in food poisoning, food manufacturers must take responsibility for food hygiene practices, from farm to fork, along complex and lengthening supply chains.

Priorities

⇨ To ensure public health is protected, government and producers need to stop seeing food as bulk industrial products and enforce welfare, traceability and food safety standards throughout their supply chains.

⇨ Consumers should be able to trust that their food is safe. In the absence of that trust, clear and consistent messages from producers and government are needed to help consumers prepare and cook food safely.

⇨ The above information is reprinted with kind permission from the Food Ethics Council. Visit www. foodethicscouncil.org for more information.

© Food Ethics Council

Food in schools

Progress in implementing the new school food standards.

In October 1999 the Government established the National Healthy Schools Programme: interim food-based standards were established for school lunches. These were later extended to include all other food provided for pupils. They first came into force in primary schools, and in 2009 for secondary schools, special schools and pupil referral units.

One aspect of the strategy has been to target a range of initiatives on 70 'spearhead' local areas which are in the bottom fifth nationally in terms of indicators of health and deprivation. This survey focused on 39 schools in 20 of those areas: 17 primary, 16 secondary, five special schools and one pupil referral unit. The survey examined how effectively the schools were promoting healthy food choices among their pupils, and the extent to which they were meeting the mandatory final food-based and, in September 2008, the final food-based and nutrient-based standards for school lunches and food-based standards for food other than lunches. It also considered how well schools related their approach to food to their work on healthy living in general.

Of the schools visited, 15 primary schools, eight secondary schools and the pupil referral unit were complying with, or close to complying with, the final food-based and nutrient-based standards for lunches: 24 of the 39 schools in total. More of the primary than the secondary schools complied with the standards for lunches, possibly because the requirements for primary schools have been in place for longer. Overall, 21 schools met the food-based standards for food other than lunches. These included ten primary schools, eight secondary schools, two special schools and the pupil referral unit. 32 of the schools had achieved National Healthy Schools Status and two were working towards the enhancement model.

The standard most often not met in primary schools was the requirement to provide a portion of fruit for every pupil eating a school lunch. In secondary schools, the standards most often not met were those restricting the provision of meat products, deep-fried foods and starchy foods cooked in fat or oil. Generally, this resulted from misinterpretation of the standards rather than deliberate non-compliance.

The most successful provision was found in the areas where the local authorities and their partners, particularly the primary health care trusts, shared a vision for improvement and had developed well-defined strategies. These were being implemented through effective inter-agency work at local level and ranged from authority-wide programmes to improve pupils' dental health and emotional wellbeing to collaborations with local sports clubs to promote more physical exercise.

The schools visited adopted a variety of approaches to extending pupils' understanding of healthy eating. These included cross-curricular topics, work within individual subjects, 'themed' days and practical experiences of handling and preparing food. Education outside the classroom also played a role. Pupils in some of the schools had the opportunity to work on local farms and allotments or with professional chefs to extend their skills and understanding.

The majority of the schools and caterers were also working hard to encourage greater take-up of meals through initiatives that included 'meal deals', being able to book tables at lunchtime to celebrate special events, free meals for new pupils and 'tasting' events for parents and the wider school community. Some of these schools had also succeeded in increasing the take-up of free school meals through sensitive advice and support for parents and carers.

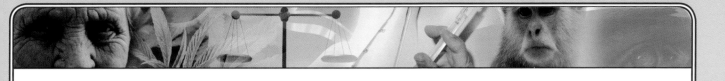

Less thought, however, had been given to providing support and advice for families who were not entitled to free school meals but whose incomes were low. Discussions with some of these parents indicated that they had to budget very carefully if they were to pay for a school meal. There were instances where siblings had to take turns to have a school lunch because of the cost.

Where unhealthy packed lunches were seen in schools, this did not necessarily reflect a lack of care and interest from parents. Their circumstances sometimes made it difficult for them to make sure that packed lunches were healthy. Lack of transport meant that they were often limited to the small range of cheap food available locally, which rarely conformed to the school's whole-school food policy. If the situation is to improve, schools, families, community representatives, local authorities and retailers need to work together to establish ways of aligning commercial and health interests. Advice and school policies on packed lunches should also suggest what food to include rather than simply focus on what to avoid.

In the schools visited, most of the pupils seen had a good understanding of what constituted a balanced diet. However, it was unclear to what extent this was influencing their choices. The most significant and consistent weakness that the survey identified was the quality of schools' monitoring of the food they provided and the impact they were having on encouraging pupils to adopt healthy diets and lifestyles.

Key findings

⇨ Of the 39 schools visited, 15 primary schools, eight secondary schools and the pupil referral unit were fully compliant or close to complying with the final food-based and nutrient-based standards for school lunches.

⇨ The food-based standards for food other than lunches were fully met in 21 of the 39 schools visited.

⇨ The most successful provision resulted from effective planning by local authorities and their partners and close collaboration between schools and a range of agencies locally.

⇨ 16 of the primary schools, 11 of the secondary schools and all the special schools visited had achieved National Healthy Schools status. Two schools were working towards the Healthy Schools enhancement model.

⇨ Almost all the schools visited had whole-school food policies which reflected varying degrees of consultation with stakeholders, monitoring and evaluation. Not all had policies on packed lunches. Where these existed, they tended to focus on what should not be included in a packed lunch rather than

providing guidance on how to provide a balanced meal in a cost-effective way.

⇨ Vegetarian options were available in all the schools visited but, in three cases, only on request. Vegetarian food was not always available as a main meal or clearly labelled.

⇨ A major weakness in the schools visited was the lack of monitoring of provision to ensure that the school food standards were fully met. Governors were often unaware of their responsibilities in this respect.

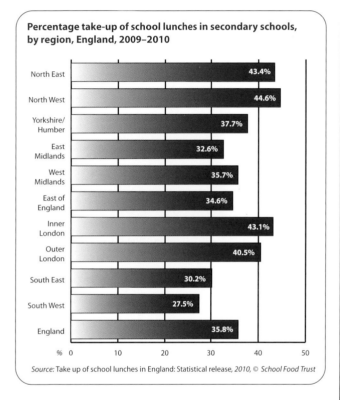

Percentage take-up of school lunches in secondary schools, by region, England, 2009–2010

Region	%
North East	43.4%
North West	44.6%
Yorkshire/Humber	37.7%
East Midlands	32.6%
West Midlands	35.7%
East of England	34.6%
Inner London	43.1%
Outer London	40.5%
South East	30.2%
South West	27.5%
England	35.8%

Source: Take up of school lunches in England: Statistical release, 2010, © School Food Trust

⇨ Most of the schools in the survey adopted a range of strategies to increase the take-up of school meals and free school meals. However, the impact of these strategies was not monitored and five of the 16 secondary schools still had systems where those entitled to free school meals could be readily identified by their peers.

⇨ The schools in the survey used a variety of ways to develop and reinforce pupils' understanding of the relationships between diet, exercise, emotional wellbeing and healthy lifestyles. However, they were not able to show to what extent their pupils were putting such understanding into practice.

25 June 2010

⇨ The above information is an extract from the Ofsted's report *Food in schools*, and is reprinted with permission. Visit www.ofsted.gov.uk for more information.

OFSTED

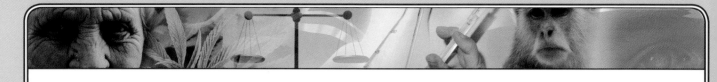

32% of pupils skip breakfast before school, study finds

Report stokes concern that children who miss morning meal are much more likely to develop chronic disease in adulthood.

By Denis Campbell

Almost a third of children regularly go without breakfast before school and are more likely than classmates to be inactive, unfit and obese, research shows.

While 68% of pupils eat before leaving home, 32% do not. Of the latter, 25% only sometimes have a morning meal and 7% never have breakfast on school days, according to findings which have raised fresh concern about children's eating habits and general health.

The study of 4,326 children, aged ten to 16, in England was reported in the *European Journal of Clinical Nutrition* and found that 26.6% of boys and 38.6% of girls skipped breakfast some or all of the time. Boys often blame lack of time, while many girls missed breakfast because they believe doing so would help them lose weight.

'We found that children who skip breakfast either occasionally or routinely are less fit, less active and more likely to be overweight or obese than those who always eat breakfast,' said lead author Dr Gavin Sandercock, a lecturer in clinical physiology at the University of Essex. 'Children with the healthiest weight were always those who regularly had breakfast before heading to school.

'These findings are worrying because we found more obesity and lower levels of physical activity among [breakfast] skippers, which is of great concern because these children are more likely to develop chronic disease in adulthood like cancer, heart disease and diabetes,' added Sandercock.

While girls who skipped breakfast are 92% more likely to become obese than female classmates who regularly eat before school, the equivalent figure in boys was 62%. But the boys were much likelier than girls to have a sedentary lifestyle and, critically, have poor cardiorespiratory (heart and lung) fitness – the best predictor of chronic illness in later life, said Sandercock.

Until now it has been thought that children who missed breakfast were more likely to be obese because they snacked during the day and ate late at night. But the study suggests that their inactive lifestyles may also play a key role.

'This research should concern parents because they are putting their children at a higher risk of being overweight unless they make sure they eat breakfast before leaving the house, and are also increasing their risk of being unfit and inactive,' said Sandercock. 'It's of great concern that 32% of parents don't do that, especially as we already know that kids' concentration and ability to learn is worse when they miss breakfast.'

> **Almost a third of children regularly go without breakfast before school and are more likely than classmates to be inactive, unfit and obese, research shows**

Professor Mitch Blair of the Royal College of Paediatrics and Child Health said: 'This is yet another study that reinforces the need for regular mealtime routines. We know that children model their behaviour on their parents and it would be interesting if the parents of the children in this study had similar habits.'

Tam Fry, founder of the Child Growth Foundation and spokesman for the National Obesity Forum, said the study underlined the importance of breakfast for everyone: 'Although 68% of the children studied always ate breakfast, there are areas of the country where, tragically, very few are given breakfast at home. That is why breakfast clubs at school are hugely important for them – not only for their physical fitness but also for their fitness to learn,' said Fry.

But Sandercock said that while breakfast clubs are a good idea, they take away from parents the responsibility of preparing food for their offspring.

The most recent NHS figures show that 22.8% of children in England starting reception year at primary school at the age of four are overweight or obese, rising to 32.6% by the time they reach year six, the last year of primary school. Previous research has also shown that children's fitness is declining worldwide, including in those who are at normal weight, and is going down faster in England than the national average.

16 August 2010

THE GUARDIAN

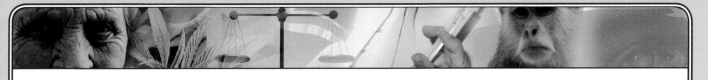

Breakfast

Lots of people claim they skip breakfast because of lack of time, or because they simply don't feel like it. But breakfast is definitely worth fitting in. No doubt you've heard the saying that 'breakfast is the most important meal of the day'. And although all our meals matter, there are a number of reasons that breakfast is really important.

Why breakfast matters

When you wake up, your body hasn't had any food for several hours. Breakfast provides the energy we need to face the day, as well as some essential vitamins and minerals. And eating breakfast could actually help you control your weight.

There is some evidence to suggest that adults and children who eat breakfast regularly are less likely to be overweight than those who don't.

Breakfast at home

For a tasty and healthy start to the day, base your breakfast on starchy foods such as bread or breakfast cereals. Try these breakfast tips and ideas:

➯ When you're choosing a breakfast cereal, try to go for one that contains wholegrains and is lower in salt and sugar. Serve your cereal with semi-skimmed, 1% or skimmed milk, or low-fat yoghurt (but remember 1% or skimmed milk isn't suitable for children under five).

➯ Try to fit in some fruit – fresh, frozen, tinned or dried fruit all count towards your five daily portions of fruit and veg. Put slices of banana on your toast, or add chunks of apple, berries or dried fruit to your cereal.

➯ Wash down your breakfast with some fruit juice – this will count as one of your fruit and veg portions, as long as it's 100% juice. A glass (150ml) of fruit juice counts as a maximum of one portion a day.

➯ Make your toast with wholemeal or granary bread. And use just a small amount of low-fat spread and some jam or marmalade. Choose a spread that is high in polyunsaturates or monounsaturates (both types of unsaturated fat), instead of one that's high in saturated fat, such as butter. Having unsaturated instead of saturated fat can help to lower your cholesterol.

➯ Why not try a fruit smoothie? If you have time, you could make it the night before and store it in the fridge, or prepare all the ingredients ready to buzz in a blender in the morning. Use fresh fruit such as banana and strawberries and some plain low-fat yoghurt or milk.

Try adding some wholegrain cereal for extra fibre. Or puree a few canned apricot halves with some orange juice.

➯ Porridge oats are cheap and contain lots of vitamins, minerals and fibre. Make your porridge with semi-skimmed or skimmed milk, or water. If you add salt to your porridge, try to get out of the habit. Add a few dried apricots or a sliced banana for extra flavour instead.

➯ For a change from ordinary toast, try a wholemeal English muffin or some toasted fruit bread.

➯ When you have more time, why not have a poached egg and mushrooms on toast? Fry the mushrooms in a non-stick pan with just a small amount of vegetable oil.

➯ If you have kids, try to have breakfast together when you can. This will help encourage them to eat breakfast.

➯ When you have time, it's fun for kids to help make their own breakfast – you could keep different cereals in the cupboard that they can mix together in a bowl. And try to have a variety of foods they can sprinkle on top, such as raisins, nuts and dried banana.

➯ An occasional full English breakfast can be part of a healthy balanced diet – just try not to have one too often.

Breakfast on the go

If you're really short of time in the mornings, you don't have to miss out. Here are some tips on how you can still fit in a healthy breakfast:

➯ Try making a packed breakfast the night before and putting it in the fridge. You could have a cheese sandwich made with a wholemeal roll, low-fat spread and a small wedge of cheese.

➯ Keep a stock of foods that are quick to grab on your way out in the morning, such as apples, pears, satsumas and bananas, mini bags of dried fruit and nuts, cartons of fruit juice and slices of fruit bread.

➯ If you work in an office, keep a box of wholegrain cereal, a bowl and a spoon at work, then you only have to pick up some milk on the way to enjoy breakfast at your desk.

➯ Try making a big fruit salad for dessert after your evening meal: then you can save what's left in a plastic box and take it with you in the morning.

➯ Crackers and breakfast bars can also be convenient if you're on the go, but bear in mind that these can be high in fat, salt and/or sugar, so remember to check the label before buying.

➯ Information from the Food Standards Agency. Visit www.eatwell.gov.uk for more.

© Crown Copyright

FOOD STANDARDS AGENCY

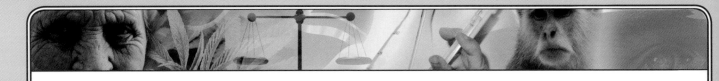

Junk food fills children's lunchboxes

Children's lunchboxes remain full of unhealthy food, new research from Leeds University shows.

By Rebecca Smithers

The infamous Turkey Twizzler may have disappeared from the school canteen, but children who eat packed lunches are still eating junk food – supplied by their parents – according to new research published today.

British children eat 5.5 billion packed lunches each year, but research from the University of Leeds shows that only 1% of their lunchboxes meet the tough nutritional standards that have been set for their classmates on school meals. The findings were described as 'appalling' by children's health campaigners, who want all children to be given free, nutritious school meals.

About half of all children in England take a packed lunch to school. In the first study of its kind, the Leeds research team, commissioned by the Government's food watchdog, the Food Standards Agency, found that 82% of their lunchboxes contained foods high in saturated fat, salt and sugar, with items chosen by parents including crisps, sweets and biscuits. Only one in five packed lunches contained any vegetables or salad and about half included an item of fruit – yet in the overwhelming majority of cases, even these fell well below the standards demanded of school dinners.

The first statutory school meal standards were introduced in 2006 due to growing evidence linking poor health in adults with obesity or poor diet in childhood. They limit the amount of foods high in salt, sugar and fats that can be served and stipulate that school meals must provide a third of the daily requirement of every nutrient for health. And although the schools watchdog, Ofsted, says schools must have a policy on packed lunches, there is no legislative imperative for them to comply with the same nutritional standards that are applied in the canteen.

Fewer than half of children's packed lunches met the Government's 2008 nutrient standards, including levels of vitamin A, folate, iron and zinc. On average, girls tended to be given more healthy foodstuffs than boys, and children at schools with fewer pupils eligible for free school meals had healthier packed lunches. Overall, the food least likely to be eaten when provided was fruit, while that most likely to be eaten was confectionery.

The research is published online today, ahead of publication in the *Journal of Epidemiology and Community Health*. It was led by Charlotte Evans of the Leeds Institute of Genetics, Health and Therapeutics, who said: 'The lack of equivalent food standards for packed lunches gives cause for concern that they will continue to lag behind the nutritional quality of school meals.'

Even without legislation, there is plenty that schools, parents and manufacturers can do to improve the situation. Evans went on: 'Our research has shown that some small steps in the right direction would make a big difference. Even if schools had a policy to provide water for children eating packed lunches, this would significantly reduce their sugar intake from sweetened drinks.

'It is important that schools support health-promotion programmes, and strategies are in place to help parents meet nutritional standards by encouraging them to include healthy foods such as protein-rich sandwiches and fruit and vegetables. Simply concentrating on restricting the junk content of lunchboxes can be counter-productive – children at schools where crisps are restricted, for example, end up with lunchboxes containing more confectionery.'

Evans added: 'We also need food manufacturers to offer better choices than the traditional high-salt, high-sugar products that busy families rely on to fill the school lunchbox on a daily basis.'

Professor Janet Cade, head of the Nutritional Epidemiology Group at Leeds, added: 'While we absolutely understand that many children prefer to take packed lunches to school, it is clear that they are not getting the same benefit from their midday meal as their classmates on school dinners. The poor quality of these meals could have serious implications for levels of childhood obesity and its long-term consequences.'

The Children's Food Campaign coordinator, Jackie Schneider, commented: 'Although these findings are appalling, we are not surprised. A whole industry has grown up around producing foods for lunchboxes, which can contain high levels of salt, fat or sugar. Parents are often misled by marketing for these lunchbox products, which make health claims like "high in vitamins" but also turn out to be high in salt, fat or sugar as well.'

Schneider concluded: 'There is now an even stronger case for giving all children a free healthy school meal, which really will start to change our food culture.'

12 January 2010

THE GUARDIAN

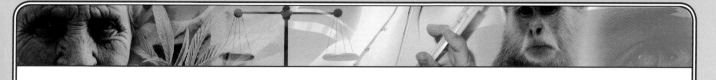

Buy healthier food

It's easy to miss the nutritional information displayed on most food packets sold in the UK. But pay attention to these labels, and they can be the key to a healthier diet.

Take a look at any food label and you'll see a list of ingredients. The ingredients list is given in order of weight, so the main ingredients in the packaged food always come first. That means that if the first few ingredients are high-fat ingredients, such as cream, butter or oil, then the food in question is high-fat food.

Most food labels also contain a nutritional analysis panel. This will usually tell you how many calories there are in a single portion and also how many calories are contained in 100 grams. If you're trying to lose weight, then it's especially useful to know how many calories are contained in one portion of the food you're looking at. But be aware: the manufacturer's concept of a portion may be different from yours.

The nutritional analysis panel will also tell you the amount of fat, saturated fat, sugar and salt per 100 grams. The Food Standards Agency has issued useful guidelines to help you decide if a food is high in fat or sugar.

⇨ Low fat = less than three grams of fat per 100 grams.

⇨ High fat = more than 20 grams of fat per 100 grams.

⇨ Low sugar = less than five grams of sugar per 100 grams.

⇨ High sugar = more than 15 grams of sugar per 100 grams.

Thanks to the introduction of traffic light labels on the front of many food packets, you can find an even easier guide to fat, sugar and salt content (see below).

Remember, a healthy diet is all about balance. You can learn more about balancing your diet by reading the Food and diet section of our website (www.nhs.uk).

At the supermarket

Now you're ready to start reading labels when you shop for food.

If you're buying ready meals, check the food labels to see how your choices stack up when it comes to calories and fat, salt and sugar content. 'Healthier option' ranges are usually lower in calories and fat than standard ranges.

But remember that even 'healthier' ready meals will probably be higher in fat and calories than the home-made equivalent. If you make the meal yourself, you could save money too.

If you're looking for a snack, try swapping your regular snack for something lower in calories.

Most chocolate bars contain between 250 and 450 calories. An apple, on the other hand, is sweet, filling and typically contains just 50 calories.

Traffic light labels

Until recently, finding out the amount of fat, saturated fat, sugars and salt in packaged food meant you had to try to make sense of the information on the backs of packets. That isn't always convenient, especially if you're in a hurry.

But now, most of the big supermarkets and many food manufacturers are using a new front-of-pack food labelling system that uses traffic light colours. This gives an at-a-glance guide to the five key factors:

⇨ fat content;

⇨ saturated fat content;

⇨ sugar content;

⇨ salt content;

⇨ calories.

Red means high, amber means medium and green means low. And, because it's on the front of food packets, you can see it immediately.

But what does it mean? In short, the more green lights, the healthier the choice.

If you buy a food that has all or mostly green lights, you know straight away that it's a healthier choice. An amber light means neither high nor low, so you can eat foods with all or mostly amber lights most of the time. But a red light means the food is high in fat, salt or sugar, and these are the foods we should be cutting down on. Try to eat these foods only on occasion.

As well as using the traffic light colours, the labels tell you how many grams of total fat, saturated fat, sugars and salt there are in a serving. And if you do want more detailed nutritional information, the nutrition panels are still there on the backs of packets.

You can learn more about food labels and healthy eating in the food labels section of the Food Standards Agency's Eatwell site (www.eatwell.gov.uk/foodlabels).

⇨ Information from the Department of Health.

NHS CHOICES

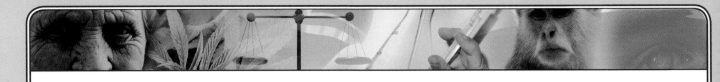

Food standards – labelling and composition

Information from the Department for Environment, Food and Rural Affairs (Defra).

Food standards legislation set out specific requirements for the labelling, composition and, in some cases, safety parameters for specific high-value foodstuffs which are potentially at risk of being misleadingly substituted with lower quality alternatives.

The legislation makes sure consumers are not misled as to the nature of a food product when it is sold to them. It also makes the playing field level for food producers, so they have established standards they can work to when producing well-known or traditional foodstuffs.

Most legislation on food standards is developed in Europe, with full involvement from UK Government officials. Secondary legislation is then used to either implement the requirements or put in place enforcement powers, depending on the nature of the European legislation. There are compositional standards in legislation for a wide variety of products. These products include bottled water, dairy, fats and oils, bread, jams and chocolate.

There are also international standards such as those produced by Codex, which, whilst they are not legally binding, are generally considered good practice. They ensure fairness in international trade and make sure consumer interests are protected.

Defra is responsible for standards legislation in England that is principally non-safety, and the Food Standards Agency (FSA) on standards that are principally safety-based.

For Scotland, Wales and Northern Ireland all domestic standards legislation is the responsibility of the FSA. The FSA has an area of their website devoted to their labelling work.

Rules covering specific compositional and labelling requirements

Bottled waters

Bottled waters are split into three categories: natural mineral water, spring water and bottled drinking water. Each has its own rules and requirements on exploitation, sale and how it is labelled.

Natural mineral waters must come from a recognised underground source and can only be subject to very limited treatments. Any water labelled 'spring water' must come from an underground source and meet certain exploitation and labelling requirements, but does not need to be from an officially recognised source. Bottled

drinking water can come from any water source and has fewer labelling restrictions than the other two categories.

Milk products

For milk products, there are legal standards that set out compositional and labelling requirements and also protect the use of dairy terms when marketing foods. Specific legal standards exist on the composition and labelling of ice cream, cream, casein and caseinates, certain UK cheeses and condensed/dried milk. The use of terms such as milk, cheese, cream, yogurt etc are also protected, so they may only be used for the associated dairy products and not misused to describe non-dairy produce.

[Food standards] legislation makes sure consumers are not misled as to the nature of a food product when it is sold

---

Meat products

For a range of meat products there is legislation setting out specific compositional and labelling requirements. The rules set out minimum meat content requirements for certain meat products sold using reserved descriptions such as sausages, burgers, corned beef, meat pies, pasties, etc. In addition, there are very specific labelling rules for certain meat products that look like a cut, joint, slice, portion or carcase of meat, where any added water over certain limits as well as any added ingredients of different animal species to the rest of the meat must be mentioned in the name of the food.

Fat and oils

Legal standards on composition for fats and oil exist for labelling them as an ingredient 'vegetable oil/fat'. In addition there are very specific rules on the labelling and composition of spreadable fats, such as butter and margarine. These set out permitted fat ranges for each type of spreadable fat: dairy spreads made with milk fat; fat spreads made with vegetable fats; and blended spreads which contain a mix of both types of fat. The legal name for a particular spread must appear prominently on packaging.

Bread and flour

The Bread and Flour Regulations 1998 lay down specific labelling and compositional standards for the breads and flours to which they apply. They also continue

DEFRA

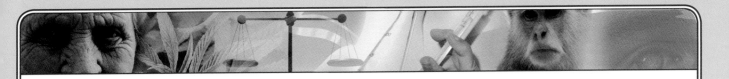

with a long-standing national requirement to restore to all flour, except wholemeal, certain vitamins and minerals such as niacin, thiamin, iron and calcium to flour manufactured and sold in the UK. They also define terms like wholemeal and self-raising.

Cocoa and chocolate products

Certain cocoa and chocolate products must comply with the reserved descriptions set out in the Cocoa and Chocolate Products Regulations 2003. The rules lay down the composition of chocolate and products including setting minimum ingredient requirements and specific labelling requirements. The amount of cocoa solids and milk solids that must be present are stipulated, as well as allowing only certain additional ingredients to be added. A cocoa solids declaration such as X% minimum is required for most chocolate products covered by the rules and also, where appropriate, a milk solids declaration is required. This enables consumers to make informed decisions about the type of chocolate they want to purchase. If you use one of the reserved descriptions covered in the regulation then your product must be made according to the defined compositional criteria.

Soluble coffee

Instant coffee is controlled by rules covered in The Coffee Extracts and Chicory Extracts (England) Regulations 2000. These define soluble coffee extracts and chicory extracts in terms of their coffee and chicory content and also provide for rules on their labelling.

Fish names

Rules are in place to make sure fish is labelled correctly and consistently at the point of sale, so purchasers know exactly what they are buying. The rules require information on:

⇨ the commercial designation of the species (i.e. an agreed common name for the species of fish);

⇨ the production method (i.e. whether caught at sea, caught in inland waters or farmed);

⇨ the catch area (i.e. either the ocean area, or in the case of freshwater fish, the country in which it was caught or farmed).

Updated rules in the form of The Fish Labelling Regulations 2010 have recently come into force which add new commercial designations (the names of fish) for species of fish that have recently come onto the market and give extra options for some others that were already listed.

Fruit juices and nectars

Detailed rules on what constitutes fruit juice are contained in the Fruit Juice and Fruit Nectars (England) Regulations 2003. These rules define terms such as fruit juice, fruit juice from concentrate, concentrated fruit juice and fruit nectar. The Regulations also authorise specific ingredients to be added to fruit juices and allow certain treatments and substances to be used, such as enzymes. In certain cases, where ingredients have been added then these must be labelled in accordance with the rules. If you use one of the reserved descriptions then your product must be made according to the defined compositional criteria.

Honey

Honey composition and labelling is controlled by the Honey (England) Regulations 2003 as amended. This legislation lays down reserved descriptions that must be used which relate to the source from which the honey is obtained (e.g. blossom, honeydew), or the processes by which it is extracted (e.g. drained) and also the way it is presented (e.g. comb, chunk honey). The Regulations lay down detailed specifications honey must comply to in terms of its composition and also set out some general quality criteria for honey. In addition, the Regulations contain some specific labelling requirements, including a requirement for country of origin labelling on honey where appropriate. If you use one of the reserved descriptions then your product must be made according to the defined compositional criteria.

Jams and marmalade

Jam and similar products must comply with the reserved descriptions as set out in the Jam and Similar Products (England) Regulations 2003. These include compositional requirements such as minimum fruit and sugar requirements and specific labelling requirements such as labelling the amount of fruit and sugar in a jam or marmalade. Products covered include jam, extra jam, jellies and marmalades. In addition, only certain ingredients are allowed to be added. The Regulations also provide national rules for mincemeat and fruit curds. If you use one of the reserved descriptions then your product must be made according to the defined compositional criteria.

Sugars

Regulations exist which lay down reserved descriptions for certain types of sugar products sold as such to the final consumer. These rules set out specifications for the sugar products covered and in some cases provide for additional labelling requirements. Products covered by the rules include white sugars, dextrose, glucose syrups and fructose.

8 November 2010

⇨ The above information is reprinted with kind permission from the Department of Environment, Food and Rural Affairs. Visit www.defra.gov.uk for more.

DEFRA

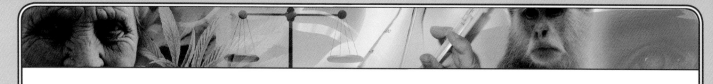

Food additives

Information from Sense about Science.

Sense About Science has been receiving an increasing number of enquiries from journalists, researchers and the general public about food additives and health. We have asked some of the specialists who help us on these subjects to provide some straightforward answers about the science behind food preservation, the meaning and reasons for E-numbers in food and drink, what scientists say about possible adverse health effects of specific additives, and how they are tested and regulated for public safety.

What are food additives?

Additives are ingredients used in the preparation of processed foods. Some of these are extracted from naturally occurring materials, others are manufactured by the chemical industry. But like every other component of food, all additives are chemicals. Preservatives, colours and flavours are the best known additives but antioxidants, emulsifiers, stabilisers, gelling agents, thickeners and sweeteners are also commonly used. The most important additives are preservatives, without which food would quickly go bad.

John Emsley, chemical scientist

What is an E-number?

Since 1986, food additives – colours, preservatives, antioxidants, stabilisers, gelling agents, thickeners, etc – have been identified on food labels, either by name or by E-number. An E-number says that it has been approved for its intended use across the European Union. Approval depends on scientific testing and monitoring and is reviewed in the light of new scientific information. Additives have been around for centuries. Nitrites and nitrates (E249–252) have been used as curing agents. Baking powder (bicarbonate of soda [sodium hydrogen carbonate], cream of tartar [potassium hydrogen tartrate, monopotassium tartrate, E336] and starch) is a 19th-century additive. Pickling is an ancient method of preservation that uses vinegar (acetic acid, E260) to prevent microbial spoilage.

Many agents that are essential for commercial food preparation and storage have their analogues in the kitchen. Caramel (E150a), a colouring agent, can be made at home by heating sugar. Gelling agents include pectin (methylated ester of galacturonic acid, E440) for jams. Preservatives include benzoic acid (E210), present in high quantities in cranberries. Some additives are clearly beneficial: in 1941 calcium was added to flour to prevent rickets; and antioxidants (necessary to prevent the fats in all prepared foods involving meat or pastry from going rancid) include ascorbic acid (vitamin C, E300) and the tocopherols (vitamin E, E306–309).

Paul Illing, toxicologist

Benzoic acid and food colourants

Benzoic acid is a natural chemical which is found in cranberries, bilberries, plums, cloves and cinnamon, some of which are said to be particularly beneficial on health grounds. It is added to processed foods to protect them. It does this by preventing the growth of microbes, and in particular pathogenic moulds and fungi. Even if the food colourants which were part of the new FSA study were removed from foods I would not like to see benzoic acid removed unless an equally effective chemical were to replace it. If it was simply removed then I am sure there would be an increase in cases of food poisoning among young children that might well be more harmful to them than a possible reduction in their bad behaviour.

John Emsley, chemical scientist

Food additives and children

There is an unclear link between food additives and hyperactivity. Whilst many parents report artificial colours and preservatives, triggering hyperactivity in their children, randomised controlled trials have

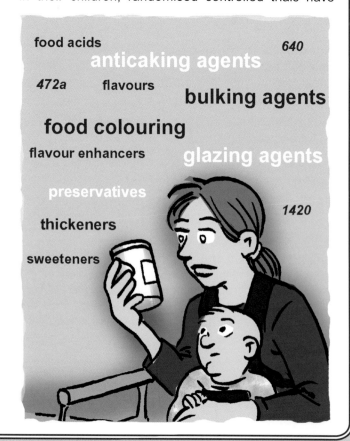

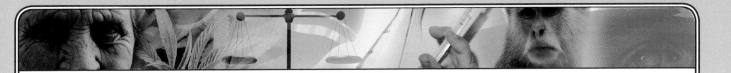

failed to demonstrate a link. A recent study carried out by Southampton University suggested that some artificial food colours, together with the preservative sodium benzoate, could have a negative effect on some children's behaviour. Whilst it is not clear which individual colours are to blame, the Food Standards Agency has suggested that parents of children showing signs of hyperactivity try eliminating the cocktail of colours investigated in this study – Sunset yellow (E110), Quinoline yellow (E104), Carmoisine (E122), Allura red (E129), Tartrazine (E102) and Ponceau 4R (E124) – to see if this leads to any benefits. It is, however, important to remember that many other factors are likely to be involved.

Sara Stanner, senior nutrition scientist

Additives cannot cause allergies but at high doses they can cause reactions or intolerances in some sensitive individuals

Some children may be susceptible to some additives and other children to different things. It is notoriously difficult to assess whether additives really affect behaviour because there are so many other confounding factors that would have to be taken into account: things like low blood sugar, tiredness and whether they had been subject to psychological stress in the time frame of the study. Asking parents to assess their children can additionally introduce the element of bias – all these factors make it very hard to look at the effect of particular additives in isolation.

Judy More, paediatric dietician

How is the use of food additives controlled?

There are EU-wide regulations that list the additives which have been tested and shown to be safe for use in food. These regulations list the foods in which each permitted additive is allowed, and its level of use. The list is first provided by the European Commission but the final decision is taken jointly by elected representatives of all EU member states and members of the European Parliament. Testing for levels of permitted additives considers differences in body weight and the needs of vulnerable members of the population, e.g. the ill, elderly. An EU-approved additive is denoted an 'E' number and can be referred to on packs as this or by its full name.

Safety tests

Safety tests include animals being given the additive, mixed with their diet, at much higher concentrations than

will occur in human food. The tests are designed to give information on any possible effects from short-term or long-term exposure to the proposed additive, including whether it may have any potential to cause cancer, affect reproductive processes or the development of the embryo or fetus if consumed by a pregnant woman. Tests are also carried out to assess its ability to interfere with genetic material in the body, which could lead to the development of cancer or adverse effects in future generations.

The results of the safety tests are assessed by independent experts (now European Food Safety Authority, EFSA) and used to calculate the Acceptable Daily Intake (ADI) for humans. The ADI is defined as 'an estimate of the amount of the food additive, expressed on a body weight basis, that can be ingested daily over a lifetime without appreciable health risk' and is expressed on a milligram per kilogram bodyweight per day basis (mg/kg bw/day). The ADI concept is used extensively by regulatory bodies throughout the world, such as the US Food and Drugs Administration (FDA), the World Health Organization (WHO) and the European Community (EC), to confirm that ingestion of all additives remains within safe levels. It applies to people of all ages, children as well as adults. After approval, additives are subject to continuous monitoring and review.

Can additives lead to allergies/intolerances?

Additives cannot cause allergies but at high doses they can cause reactions or intolerances in some sensitive individuals. But the number of people suffering a reaction is small when investigated by randomised controlled trials (RCTs), and much rarer than an allergy/intolerance to a natural food.

Are there banned additives?

Yes, some additives that were approved for use have been withdrawn from the food supply (e.g. E103, E105) because the safety tests on them are constantly reviewed.

How are dietary intakes of food additives monitored?

Food surveillance studies looking at levels in samples of foods and using national data (e.g. National Diet and Nutrition Survey, NDNS) to estimate intake in highest consumers versus ADI were carried out in the UK by the Ministry of Agriculture, Fisheries and Food (MAFF) and now by the FSA. The FSA are responsible for monitoring their use and taking appropriate steps to ensure that intake does not exceed recommended levels. Reports on intakes are also published by the European Commission.

SENSE ABOUT SCIENCE

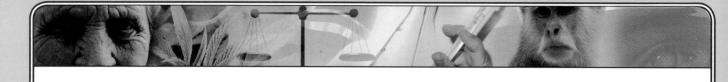

Why do medicines containing some artificial colourings carry health warnings when foods containing the same additives do not?

The labelling of additives in medicines and foods is controlled by different legislation (the information on additive health warnings on medical products is published by the European Commission in *Guidelines for medicinal products for human use* – excipients in the label and package leaflet of medicinal products for human use). Medicines need to alert consumers of any possible reactions to any of their ingredients. However, as there is no evidence that our intakes of these additives from foods and drinks cause any problems for the majority of the population, health warnings on foods and drinks are unwarranted.

Sara Stanner, senior nutrition scientist

Additives are ingredients used in the preparation of processed foods. Some of these are extracted from naturally occurring materials, others are manufactured by the chemical industry

---

The cocktail effect

Concern has been expressed about the multiplicative or 'cocktail' effect. Safety tests look at the effects of levels of one additive. Although less is known about the cumulative effect of exposure to multiple additives, chemically speaking, such effects are rare and scientifically well-understood. What the cocktail description usually implies is that, while individual substances may be considered safe at current levels of exposure, they may interact with each other and create unforeseen effects. But the natural world is a 'cocktail of chemicals' so our bodies are used to dealing with a mix of substances. The same processes of storing, neutralising, breaking down and excreting occur when we encounter new substances.

Food additives are not a new phenomenon

For centuries people have enhanced their food with naturally available flavourings, preservatives and dyes. With our increasingly complex food supply, food additives play a vital role. Never before has the range and choice of foods been so wide either in supermarkets, specialist food shops or when eating out. As consumers we are demanding more variety, choice and convenience alongside higher standards of safety and wholesomeness at affordable prices. Meeting these consumer expectations can only be achieved using modern food processing technologies which include the use of a variety of food additives proven effective and safe through long use and rigorous testing. Without additives bread would become stale very quickly, fatty foods would turn rancid and most tinned fruits and vegetables would lose their firmness and colour. Even organic foods can contain additives – currently 29 additives are approved for use in organic foods.

Nigel Denby, nutrition consultant

⇨ The above information is reprinted with kind permission from Sense About Science. Visit www.senseaboutscience.org.uk for more information.

© *Sense About Science*

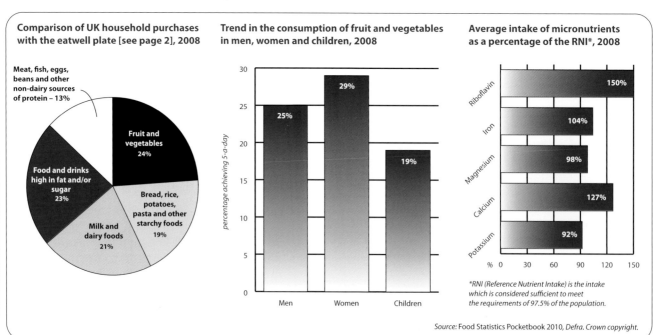

Comparison of UK household purchases with the eatwell plate [see page 2], 2008

Meat, fish, eggs, beans and other non-dairy sources of protein – 13%
Fruit and vegetables 24%
Food and drinks high in fat and/or sugar 23%
Bread, rice, potatoes, pasta and other starchy foods 19%
Milk and dairy foods 21%

Trend in the consumption of fruit and vegetables in men, women and children, 2008

percentage achieving 5-a-day

Men 25%
Women 29%
Children 19%

Average intake of micronutrients as a percentage of the RNI*, 2008

Riboflavin 150%
Iron 104%
Magnesium 98%
Calcium 127%
Potassium 92%

% 0 30 60 90 120 150

*RNI (Reference Nutrient Intake) is the intake which is considered sufficient to meet the requirements of 97.5% of the population.

Source: Food Statistics Pocketbook 2010, *Defra. Crown copyright.*

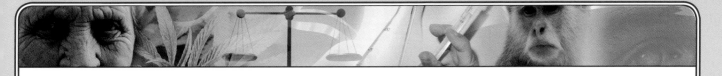

Healthy eating habits uncovered

Healthy eating is an important issue for contemporary society and is communicated through many different initiatives and campaigns today in the UK.

Let's look at two pieces of advice recommended for leading a healthy lifestyle and how British shoppers are changing their behaviour as a result.

Eating five portions of fruit and vegetables a day

According to our recent research, more than two-fifths (43%) of shoppers say they eat five portions of fruit or vegetables a day as part of a healthy lifestyle. The figure has been steadily increasing since 2006 when less than a third (32%) of shoppers made the claim. Those in the lower social grades, however, are not responding to the five-a-day message.

⇨ Only 26% of shoppers from social grades DE claim to meet the five-a-day target – showing no increase at all over the last four years.

⇨ While 50% of ABs and 48% of C1C2s consume five portions of fruit or vegetables a day.

⇨ The biggest increase over the past 12 months is among shoppers in social grade C2, up 25 percentage points.

When asked about activities that they follow to lead a healthy lifestyle, eating five-a-day was the most popular answer:

⇨ 43% said they eat five-a-day (compared with 32% in 2006).

⇨ 40% said they drink more water (38% in 2006).

⇨ 38% said they eat low-fat versions of food (33% in 2006).

⇨ 24% said they are cutting down on their salt intake (19% in 2006).

⇨ Just over a third (36%) of shoppers said that they intend to take more exercise – a figure which has been static since 2006 (35%).

The food industry has got behind the five-a-day campaign and helped to make it a success. It is clear that the messages underlining the importance of eating five-a-day are getting through to the British shopper, but the Government, the food industry and other stakeholders need to continue to work together to keep pushing the message to the general public.

Eating breakfast

Nutritionally, breakfast is of vital importance, providing us with the energy needed for the day ahead, and vitamins and minerals for overall good health. Breakfast is often regarded as the most important meal of the day and NHS campaigns have focused on linking a nutritious breakfast with a healthy diet. Breakfast also plays a key role in helping to tackle obesity.

So, we asked British shoppers whether or not they had breakfast during the week and at weekends and the results were surprising.

⇨ 27% of shoppers miss breakfast at some stage during the week.

⇨ Despite a recent campaign by the NHS, 'Breakfast4life', more than a quarter (27%) of shoppers miss breakfast at some stage during the week, up from one in five (19%) in 2004. One in six (16%) never have breakfast, compared to one in eight (12%) six years ago.

⇨ At the weekends, 21% are missing breakfast, up from 15% in 2004. There has been a similar increase in the proportion missing breakfast on weekdays.

⇨ Interestingly, there is a difference between men and women, with around a fifth of women (23%) skipping breakfast compared to around three in ten men (31%).

⇨ The research also found that shoppers aged 15 to 24, and those working, are least likely to have breakfast.

↳ A third (33%) of 15- to 24-year-olds miss breakfast during weekdays, compared to 22% in 2004.

↳ 32% of those working miss breakfast at some stage during the week, compared to 20% of non-workers.

So why are people still missing breakfast? Are they unaware of its importance or are there other reasons?

Our research revealed that work and time pressures are resulting in more people skipping breakfast and prioritising other things over this important meal. Survey respondents cited factors such as 'catching up on sleep' and 'getting ready for work' as more important than eating breakfast. Many mothers recognised the importance of ensuring their children ate breakfast, but would actually skip breakfast themselves due to time pressures.

Opportunities for retailers and manufacturers

It is clear that although the food industry supports the healthy eating message, more needs to be done to communicate its different aspects.

INSTITUTE OF GROCERY DISTRIBUTION

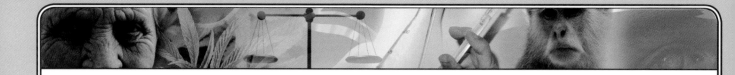

Building awareness of five-a-day and eating breakfast will continue to be important and there are significant opportunities for retailers and manufacturers to provide time-saving solutions that also meet shoppers' budget constraints. Our industry should continue to innovate in the variety, quality and convenience of these ranges for all meal occasions.

⇨ The above information is reprinted with the kind permission of the Institute of Grocery Distribution (IDG). Visit www.igd.com/healthyeatinghabits to view this article online.

Top doctor calls for urgent action on salt and fats in food

Lindsey Davies says minimum health standards should be imposed if the food industry does not cut 'irresponsible' amounts of fat and salt in products.

By Denis Campbell

One of Britain's top doctors has accused the food industry of being 'profoundly irresponsible' for adding unhealthy amounts of fat and salt to its products.

Lindsey Davies, the new president of the UK Faculty of Public Health, wants ministers to bring in legal minimum health standards for food if manufacturers do not undertake dramatic action to strip out harmful ingredients such as transfats and excess salt. Both are added during production and have been implicated in causing tens of thousands of deaths a year through strokes and heart attacks.

'The food industry should be about producing food, and food is a basic requirement of a healthy, productive life and wellbeing. Adding things to food that reduce health and wellbeing, such as transfats or too much salt, strikes me as profoundly irresponsible,' said Davies, who represents 3,500 public health doctors in the NHS, local government and academia. 'Overall, I think it is profoundly disappointing that the food industry hasn't taken its responsibilities more seriously.'

The links between unhealthy food and conditions such as heart disease, strokes, obesity and some cancers mean action is urgently needed, Davies added. Drink-driving laws, the ban on smoking in public places and the compulsory wearing of seatbelts show that the Government sometimes has to intervene in order to protect people from health harms, she said.

While some supermarkets have made commendable progress in improving product recipes to make them healthier, too many have done too little, Davies said. New laws to ban unhealthily high levels of salt, transfats and saturated fats would be necessary without major progress by industry, she added.

It was 'very odd' that there are not already legal health and safety standards for food, she said. 'Unhealthy food is a major health problem in this country,' Davies said.

The Food and Drink Federation, which represents major producers and retailers, hit back. Barbara Gallani, its director of food safety and science, said Davies was 'out of touch with what the industry has been achieving' in terms of reformulation. For example, transfats have been virtually eliminated and some firms have cut the amount of salt in products such as soups, cereals, biscuits and cakes, in some cases by up to 50%, in the last five years, said Gallani. Such a move would also deny consumers choice in their eating habits, she added.

The Food Standards Agency advises adults not to consume more than 6g of salt a day. Average intake fell from 9.5g to 8.6g between 2000 and 2008, an FSA spokesman said. Intake of transfats – man-made substances used to bulk out food or give it a longer shelf-life – is about 1% of total food energy intake, about half of what the World Health Organization recommends, he added.

Senior doctors backed Davies's call. Steve Field, chair of the Royal College of GPs, said: 'Ready meals are a particular problem for both salt and transfats. Manufacturers should look at themselves in the mirror and realise the harms they are doing to other human beings.' Terence Stephenson, president of the Royal College of Paediatrics and Child Health, said: 'Given that one-third of our children are overweight or obese, tackling our unhealthy food culture is vital. Food advertising should be restricted, planning controls used to limit fast-food premises near places where young people congregate and the price of food examined to find ways to make healthier products more affordable.'

7 July 2010

INSTITUTE OF GROCERY DISTRIBUTION / THE GUARDIAN

Obesity and the economics of prevention: fit not fat

Obesity is becoming public health enemy number one in most OECD countries. Severely obese people die eight to ten years sooner than those of normal-weight, similar to smokers, with every 15 extra kilograms increasing risk of early death by approximately 30%. In ten European countries, research shows that obesity doubles the odds of being unable to live a normal active life.

Obesity is expensive, and a burden on health systems. Throughout their lives, health care expenditures for obese people are at least 25% higher than for someone of normal weight and increase rapidly as people get fatter. However, the reduction in life expectancy is so great that obese people incur lower health care costs over their lifetime (13% less, according to a Dutch study) than those of normal weight, but more than smokers, on average. Obesity is estimated to be responsible for 1% to 3% of total health expenditure in most countries (5% to 10% in the United States) and costs will rise rapidly in coming years as obesity-related diseases set in.

What are the trends in obesity – past and future?

Until 1980, fewer than one in ten people were obese. Since then, rates have doubled or tripled and in almost half of OECD countries one in two people is now overweight or obese. If recent trends continue, projections suggest that more than two out of three people will be overweight or obese in some OECD countries within the next ten years.

Height and weight have been increasing since the 18th century, as income, education and living conditions gradually improved over time. While weight gains were largely beneficial to the health and longevity of our ancestors, an alarming number of people have now crossed the line beyond which further gains are dangerous.

Who is affected by obesity and what are the social impacts?

Women are more often obese than men, but male obesity rates have been growing faster than female rates in most OECD countries.

Obesity is more common among the poor and the less educated. In several OECD countries, women with little education are two to three times more likely to be overweight than more educated women, but smaller or no disparities exist for men.

Social disparities are also present in children (both boys and girls) in England, France and the United States, but not in Korea.

Children who have at least one obese parent are three to four times more likely to be obese themselves. This is partly genetic, but children generally share their parents' unhealthy diets and sedentary lifestyles, an influence which has played an important role in the spread of obesity.

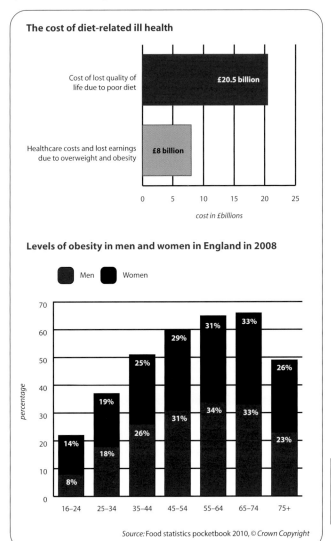

The cost of diet-related ill health

Cost of lost quality of life due to poor diet — £20.5 billion

Healthcare costs and lost earnings due to overweight and obesity — £8 billion

cost in £billions

Levels of obesity in men and women in England in 2008

■ Men ■ Women

percentage

Age	Men	Women
16–24	14%	8%
25–34	19%	18%
35–44	25%	26%
45–54	29%	31%
55–64	31%	34%
65–74	33%	33%
75+	26%	23%

Source: Food statistics pocketbook 2010, © Crown Copyright

OECD

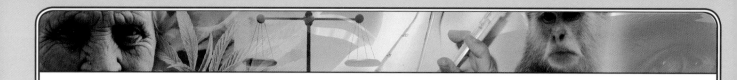

Poor health goes hand in hand with poor job prospects for many obese people. Employers prefer normal-weight over obese candidates, partly due to expectations of lower productivity. This contributes to an employment and wage gap. In the United States, more than 40% of severely obese white women are out of work compared to just over 30% for all women. Obese people earn up to 18% less than people of normal weight. They need to take more days off, claim more disability benefits and tend to be less productive on the job than people of normal weight. In northern European countries, obese people are up to three times more likely than others to receive a disability pension, and in the United States they are 76% more likely to suffer short-term disability. When production losses are added to health care costs, obesity accounts for over 1% of GDP in the United States.

How did obesity become a problem?

There is no one smoking gun which explains the obesity epidemic. Instead, a series of changes, harmless by themselves, have massed into a slow-burning catastrophe. Increased food supply, combined with major changes in food production and constant sophisticated use of promotion and persuasion, have cut the price of calories dramatically and made convenience foods all too available. At the same time, changing working and living conditions mean that fewer people prepare traditional meals from raw ingredients. Less physical activity at work, more women in the labour force, higher levels of stress and job insecurity and longer working hours are all factors directly or indirectly contributing to the lifestyle changes causing the obesity epidemic.

Government policies have, inadvertently, also played a part. Examples include subsidies (e.g. in agriculture) and taxation affecting food prices; transport policies that encourage the use of private cars and make walking to work an oddity; urban planning policies that make commuting commonplace, and lead to the creation of deprived urban areas with no greengrocers, many fast food outlets and few playgrounds and sports facilities.

What can governments and markets do to promote better health?

Governments can help people change their lifestyle by making new healthy options available or by making existing ones more accessible and affordable. Alternatively, they can use persuasion, education and information to make healthy options more attractive. This gentle approach is more expensive, hard to deliver and hard to monitor. A tougher approach, through regulation and fiscal measures, is more transparent but it hits all consumers indiscriminately, so can have high political and welfare costs. It may also be difficult to organise and enforce and have regressive effects.

A survey of national policies covering OECD and other EU countries shows that governments are stepping up efforts to promote a culture of healthy eating and active living. Most have initiatives aimed at school-age children, such as changes in school meals and vending machines, better facilities for physical activity and health education. Many also disseminate nutrition guidelines and health promotion messages such as encouraging 'active transport' – cycling and walking – and active leisure. Governments are reluctant to use regulation and fiscal levers because of the complex regulatory process, the enforcement costs and the likelihood of confrontation with key industries.

If recent trends continue, projections suggest that more than two out of three people will be overweight or obese in some OECD countries within the next ten years

The private sector, including employers, the food and beverage industry, the pharmaceutical industry and the sports industry have a role to play. Governments are demanding that the food and beverage industry take action: reformulate food production to avoid particularly unhealthy ingredients (e.g. saturated fats and too much salt), reduce excessive portion sizes and provide healthy menu alternatives; limit advertising, particularly to vulnerable groups like children; and inform consumers about food contents.

Which interventions work best and at what cost?

Government actions to tackle obesity – health education and promotion, regulation and fiscal measures and lifestyle counselling by family doctors – are a better investment than many treatments currently provided by OECD health care systems. Combining these interventions in a comprehensive prevention strategy, targeting different age groups and determinants of obesity, would provide an affordable and cost-effective solution, significantly enhancing overall health gains relative to isolated actions. The price of countering obesity would be as low as US$12 per capita in Mexico, US$19 in Japan and England, US$22 in Italy and US$32 in Canada. This is a tiny fraction of health expenditure in those countries, and a small proportion of the 3% of their healthcare budgets that OECD countries now spend on prevention. A comprehensive strategy would prevent, every year, 155,000 deaths from chronic diseases in Japan, 75,000 in Italy, 70,000 in England, 55,000 in Mexico and 40,000 in Canada. It would delay or prevent the onset of chronic diseases, cutting disability

OECD

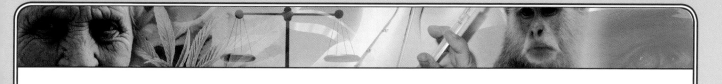

and improving quality of life. The single most effective intervention in this package is individual counselling by family doctors, although government regulation, taxes and subsidies can generate health gains at a much lower cost.

Interventions give people extra years of healthy life, reducing health care costs. They also mean, however, that people will live longer with years of life added in the oldest age groups, increasing the need for health care. The result is that effective obesity prevention policies are unlikely to greatly reduce total health expenditure and could, at best, generate reductions in the order of 1% of total expenditure for major chronic diseases. That said, the primary goal of prevention is to improve population health and longevity, and our results show that government intervention can be effective.

Can we hope for a future which is Fit, not Fat?

Just as there is no smoking gun responsible for obesity, there is no magic bullet to cure it. 20 years ago, the epidemiologist Geoffrey Rose estimated that reducing the average weight of a population by 1.25% (e.g. less than 900 grams for a person weighing 70kg) would reduce the rate of obesity by 25%. Unfortunately, none of the strategies tried so far can, alone, achieve even that small success. An effective prevention strategy must combine complementary strengths: population approaches – health promotion campaigns, taxes and

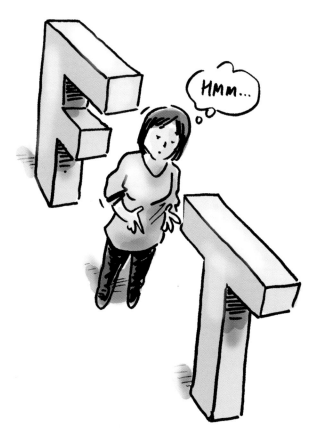

subsidies, or government regulation – with individual approaches such as counselling by family doctors to change what people perceive as the norm in healthy behaviour.

Adopting a 'multi-stakeholder' approach is a sensible way forward. Governments must retain overall control of initiatives to prevent chronic diseases and encourage private sector commitment. Because there will be conflicting interests, fighting obesity and associated chronic diseases will demand compromise and co-operation by all stakeholders. Failure would impose heavy burdens on future generations.

Summary of key facts on obesity and the economics of prevention

⇨ One in two people is now overweight or obese in almost half of OECD countries. Rates are projected to increase further and in some countries two out of three people will be obese within ten years.

⇨ An obese person incurs 25% higher health expenditures than a person of normal weight in any given year. Obesity is responsible for 1–3% of total health expenditures in most OECD countries (5–10% in the United States).

⇨ A severely obese person is likely to die eight to ten years earlier than a person of normal weight.

⇨ Poorly educated women are two to three times more likely to be overweight than those with high levels of education, but almost no disparities are found for men.

⇨ Obese people earn up to 18% less than non-obese people.

⇨ Children who have at least one obese parent are three to four times more likely to be obese.

⇨ A comprehensive prevention strategy would avoid, every year, 155,000 deaths from chronic diseases in Japan, 75,000 in Italy, 70,000 in England, 55,000 in Mexico and 40,000 in Canada.

⇨ The annual cost of such strategy would be US$12 per capita in Mexico, US$19 in Japan and England, US$22 in Italy and US$32 in Canada. The cost per life year gained through prevention is less than US$20,000 in these five countries.

23 September 2010

⇨ OECD (2010), *Obesity and the Economics of Prevention: Fit not Fat*, OECD Publishing, http://dx.doi.org/10.1787/9789264084865-en

OECD

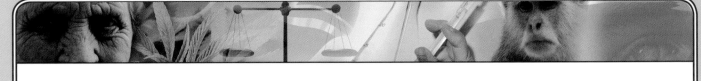

The truth about fad diets

Following the latest diet is often not a good idea if you want to lose weight and keep it off.

Below are some of the problems with many diets, plus tips on how to lose weight healthily. As well as eating healthily, it's important to be active as this burns calories and can help you lose weight.

Five reasons to avoid fad diets

Many weight loss diets promise to help you lose weight quickly. Often, these diets focus on short-term results and don't work in the long term. They may also be bad for your health.

Here are five reasons to avoid them:

⇨ Many diets, especially crash diets, involve dramatically reducing the number of calories you consume. You may lose weight quickly but you risk losing muscle rather than fat. 'Crash diets make you feel very unwell and unable to function properly,' says dietitian Ursula Arens. 'Because they are nutritionally unbalanced, crash diets can lead to long-term poor health, including eating disorders.'

Detox diets are based on the idea that toxins build up in the body and can be removed by eating, or not eating, certain things. However, there's no evidence that toxins build up in our bodies

⇨ Some diets recommend cutting out certain foods, such as meat, fish, wheat or dairy products. Cutting out certain food groups altogether could prevent you from getting important nutrients and vitamins, which your body needs to function properly.

⇨ Some diets are very low in carbohydrates (such as pasta, bread and rice), which are an essential source of energy. While you may lose weight on these types of diets, they're often high in protein and fat, which can make you ill. 'It has been suggested that the high protein content of these diets "dampens" the appetite and feelings of hunger,' says Arens. Many low-carbohydrate diets allow you to eat foods that are high in saturated fat, such as butter, cheese and meat. Too much saturated fat can raise your cholesterol and increase your risk of heart disease and stroke.

⇨ Detox diets are based on the idea that toxins build up in the body and can be removed by eating, or not eating, certain things. However, there's no evidence

that toxins build up in our bodies. If they did, we would feel very ill. 'Detox diets do not work,' says Arens. 'They are, in effect, a form of modified fasting.'

⇨ Some fad diets are based on eating a single food or meal, such as cabbage soup. Others make far-fetched claims, for example that eating grapefruit can help burn body fat. Often, there is little or no evidence to back up these claims. 'If followed over long periods, these diets are very unbalanced and bad for your health,' says Arens. 'You may lose weight in the short term, but it's much better to lose weight gradually and to be healthy.'

The healthy way to lose weight

We put on weight when the number of calories we eat over time exceeds the number of calories we burn off through normal everyday activities and exercise.

The only way to lose weight healthily and keep it off is to make permanent changes to the way you eat and

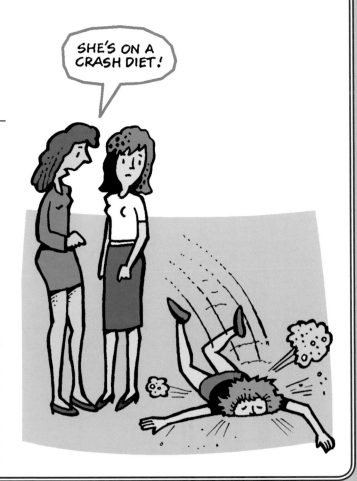

SHE'S ON A CRASH DIET!

NHS CHOICES

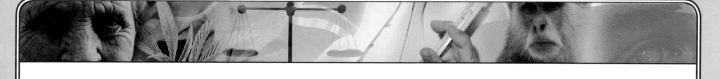

exercise. These don't have to be big changes. A few small alterations to your diet can help you achieve a healthy weight, and there are plenty of ways to make physical activity part of your everyday routine.

Aim to lose about 0.5–1kg (1–2lb) a week until you reach a healthy weight for your height. You should be able to lose this amount if you eat about 500 to 600 calories fewer a day than you need.

An average man needs about 2,500 calories a day and an average woman about 2,000 calories to stay the same weight.

> *Aim to lose about 0.5–1kg (1–2lb) a week until you reach a healthy weight for your height. You should be able to lose this amount if you eat about 500 to 600 calories fewer a day than you need*

Five ways to kick-start your healthy weight loss plan

Here are five simple things you can do to eat healthily and help you lose weight.

⇨ To reduce the amount of fat you eat, you could trim the fat off meat, drink skimmed or semi-skimmed milk instead of full fat, choose a reduced- or low-fat spread and replace cream with low-fat yoghurt.

⇨ Eat wholegrain foods, such as wholemeal bread,

brown rice and pasta. They're digested more slowly than the white varieties so will help you feel full for longer.

⇨ Don't skip breakfast. A healthy breakfast will give you the energy you need to start the day, and there's some evidence that people who eat breakfast regularly are less likely to be overweight.

⇨ If you feel like a snack, try having a drink first, such as a glass of water or cup of tea. Often we think we're hungry when really we're thirsty.

⇨ Aim to eat at least five portions of fruit and vegetables a day. Go to the '5 A DAY shopping planner' on the NHS Choices website for lots of ideas on how to get your five a day.

Fitness tips to boost your healthy weight loss

Regular exercise will not only help you lose weight but could also reduce your risk of developing a serious illness.

Adults should do at least 30 minutes of activity five times a week for general health benefits. To lose weight and keep it off, you need to do at least 60 minutes of activity regularly.

22 December 2009

⇨ Reproduced by kind permission of the Department of Health.

Activities performed by people to achieve a healthy lifestyle

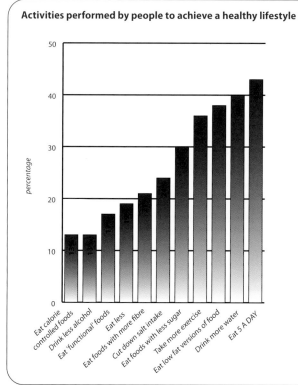

Regional household consumption of fruit and vegetables 2006-2008

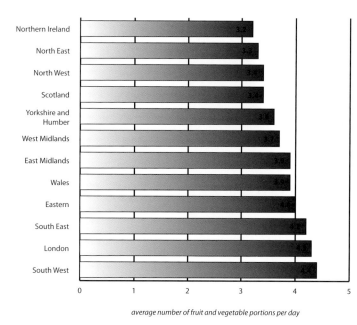

average number of fruit and vegetable portions per day

Source: Food statistics pocket handbook 2010, © Crown copyright

NHS CHOICES

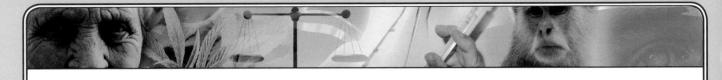

Saturated fat

We all need some fat in our diet. Fat provides essential fatty acids, it helps the body to carry and absorb fat-soluble vitamins and it also provides the body with energy.

Fat in food is made up of two different types of fatty acids: saturates and unsaturates. Unsaturated fatty acids can be either monounsaturates or polyunsaturates, depending on their chemical structure. All fats contain a combination of the two types (saturated and unsaturated), but the proportion of each varies greatly with different foods. Fats in the diet are described as 'saturated' or 'unsaturated' according to the proportions of fatty acids present. For example, butter is often described as a 'saturated fat' because it has more saturated fatty acids than unsaturated fatty acids, while most vegetable oils are described as 'unsaturated fats' as they have more mono- and polyunsaturates than saturates.

So what is the issue with saturated fat?

A high intake of fat, and in particular saturated fat, is associated with negative health consequences. Eating a diet that is high in saturated fat is associated with raised levels of blood cholesterol, which can increase the risk of developing heart disease.

In the UK, most people are eating too much saturated fat. Average intake of saturates in both men and women is approximately 13% of food energy, which is higher than the recommended target of 11%. The average man should eat no more than 30g saturated fat a day and the average woman, no more than 20g.

Which foods are high in saturated fat?

⇨ Fatty cuts of meat, poultry skin and red meat.

⇨ Meat products such as sausages and pies.

⇨ Whole milk and full-fat dairy products such as cheese and cream.

⇨ Butter, ghee and lard.

⇨ Coconut oil and palm oil.

⇨ Pastry.

⇨ Cakes and biscuits.

⇨ Sweets and chocolate.

Tips for cutting down

⇨ Read the label. Most food products state how much saturated fat is in the food. Look for 'sat fat' or 'fat of which saturates', compare similar food items and choose the option that has less saturated fat. To help you to interpret the food label:

↳ If a product contains more than 5g of saturated fat per 100g, this is considered a lot.

↳ If a product contains less than 1g of saturated fat per 100g, this is considered a little.

⇨ Choose lean cuts of meat, trim off any visible fat and remove the skin from poultry meat such as chicken or turkey.

⇨ Choose leaner types of beef mince, or try using turkey mince, which is even leaner.

⇨ Choose lower-fat or reduced-fat dairy products, such as 1% fat milk, low-fat yogurts and reduced-fat cheese.

⇨ Choose a product that contains mostly unsaturated fats as your everyday oil or fat spread rather than one that is high in saturated fats.

⇨ Choose sunflower, rapeseed or olive oils that are high in unsaturated fats for cooking and only use in small amounts.

⇨ Grill your meat rather than frying it.

⇨ Eat a balanced diet, with plenty of fruit and vegetables and starchy foods such as rice, pasta and potatoes, as these are lower in saturated fat.

⇨ Choose healthy snacks when you are on the go, such as fruit or dried fruit and nuts rather than cakes, biscuits and chocolate, which are often high in saturated fat.

Remember, we all need some fat and so it doesn't need to be cut out of the diet completely. Some polyunsaturated fatty acids that you find in oily fish, nuts, seeds and vegetable oil (rapeseed oil, sunflower oil) are essential for health and it is important that we get these fatty acids from our diet. These types of fatty acids can help protect against heart disease and, in general, unsaturated fatty acids can help to reduce our blood cholesterol levels. We should try to substitute poly- and monounsaturated fats for saturated fats rather than eating them in addition to saturated types.

⇨ The above information is reprinted with kind permission from the British Nutrition Foundation. Visit www.nutrition.org.uk for more information on this and other related topics.

© British Nutrition Foundation

BRITISH NUTRITION FOUNDATION

Salt and your health

Information from Consensus Action on Salt and Health.

Salt can damage your health

Small amounts of salt are essential for our wellbeing. Adults need less than one gram per day and children need even less, but most adults now eat between seven to ten grams per day, far more than needed. The current amounts of salt eaten in the UK can have many harmful effects on our health, and therefore reducing our salt intake is very important. Adults should consume less than six grams of salt per day and children much less.

Blood pressure is the biggest cause of death in the world through the strokes and heart attacks it causes

Blood pressure

Blood pressure is the biggest cause of death in the world through the strokes and heart attacks it causes. The higher our blood pressure, the greater our risk. Salt slowly puts up our blood pressure and eating too much is responsible for many thousands of strokes, heart attacks and heart failure deaths each year in the UK. Eating less salt lowers blood pressure and reduces the risk of heart disease and stroke. For every one gram of salt we cut from our average daily intake there would be 6,000 fewer deaths from strokes and heart attacks each year in the UK. Over a longer period of time, reducing salt intake will have an even greater effect as it will prevent the rise in blood pressure that occurs as we get older. It is particularly important that children do not eat too much salt, as blood pressure first starts to rise in childhood.

Stroke

Stroke is the leading cause of severe adult disability and the third biggest killer in the UK with an estimated 150,000 strokes and mini-strokes each year. High blood pressure is the single most important risk factor for stroke. Salt is therefore directly responsible for many of these strokes. Over 40% of all strokes could be prevented by tackling high blood pressure. There is also increasing evidence that salt may have a direct effect on strokes, independent of and in addition to the effect it has on blood pressure.

Heart attacks and heart failure

Raised blood pressure is a major risk factor for coronary heart disease, stroke and heart attacks. Coronary heart disease is the commonest cause of death in the UK. Untreated high blood pressure can also lead to heart failure, which can make the pumping action of the heart less effective. Reducing salt intake will help to prevent high blood pressure and so reduce the risk of heart attacks and heart failure.

Osteoporosis

Salt intake is the major factor controlling the amount of calcium in the urine and the amount of calcium lost from bones. As calcium is vital for bone strength, high salt intake may lead to weakening of the bones and an increased risk of osteoporosis. Osteoporosis leads to

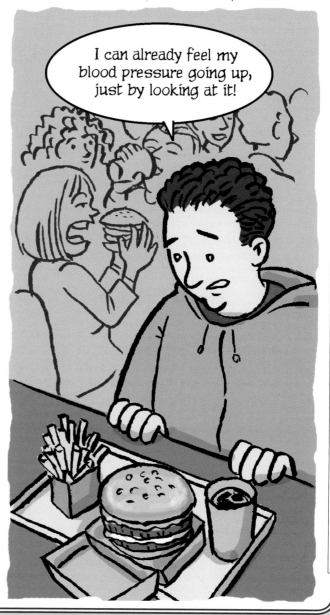

I can already feel my blood pressure going up, just by looking at it!

CONSENSUS ACTION ON SALT AND HEALTH

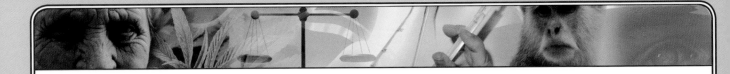

bone fractures and breakages. If we do not achieve the maximum strength of our bones when we reach our mid to late twenties, our risk of developing osteoporosis later in life is increased.

Obesity

Obesity is an increasing problem in the UK. Whilst salt is not the cause of obesity, it increases thirst and the amount of fluids consumed, particularly sweetened soft drinks. A third of all British adults, or 13 million people, will be obese by 2012 if current trends continue. A reduction in salt intake would cause a major reduction in the number of sweetened soft drinks being consumed, both by adults and children. Studies in the UK have shown that a reduction in sweetened soft drink consumption is likely to reduce the number of children developing obesity.

Stomach cancer

Salt, particularly in high concentration, damages the delicate lining of the stomach. This makes it more vulnerable to infections by *Helicobacter pylori*, a type of bacteria that causes both stomach ulcers and stomach cancer. Countries where people eat a lot of salty foods tend to have high rates of stomach cancer. In countries that have a higher salt intake than we have in the UK, for example Northern China, Japan and Korea, this is a major public health problem.

Kidney stones

Salt increases the amount of calcium in our urine. Reducing salt intake has been shown to reduce calcium excretion, and reduce reoccurrences of kidney stones, as kidney stones have calcium as their basic constituent.

Kidney disease

High blood pressure has been shown to increase the amount of protein in the urine, which is a major risk factor for the decline of kidney function, and there is increasing evidence that a high salt intake may increase how quickly kidney disease progresses where it is already present. Over three million people in the UK are at risk of Chronic Kidney Disease. In addition, the water retention that occurs with a higher salt diet will increase blood pressure, which also increases the risk of kidney disease.

Other effects of salt on our health

A reduction in salt intake may also be beneficial for keeping a number of other conditions under control, such as asthma and Ménières disease. Salt reduction is recommended for people with diabetes because keeping blood pressure in the healthy range helps to reduce your risk of the long-term complications of diabetes. A high

salt diet can also lead to water retention. Many people with water retention, including women with premenstrual water retention, find considerable improvement in their symptoms by reducing their salt intake.

Other simple reductions

Many processed and well-known-brand foods are high in salt, so try to cut down on these by both swapping for retailers' own-brand products, and switching to more fresh foods such as fish, chicken, meat, fruit and vegetables.

Labelling

Many of us now check labels for the salt content of the food we buy in supermarkets and shops. By looking at the label we can add up how much salt we are eating each day, and how much we are giving to our families. Most food labels now give the amount of salt the food contains either per 100 grams or per portion. If the label only gives the sodium content, you need to multiply sodium by 2.5 to get the salt content. 1g of sodium per 100g = 2.5g of salt per 100g. Try to think about how much of the food you will be eating. Look at the size of the packet and use this as a guide – is this more or less than 100g? From this you can work out the salt content of the portion you will eat.

Adjust to less salt

The salty taste of foods depends on the salt content of the food and also the sensitivity of the taste receptors in your mouth. Initially, when you reduce your salt intake foods tend to taste bland, but after two or three weeks your taste receptors become more sensitive, getting the same effect from lower levels of salt and you will start to taste the real delicious flavour of natural food. Give yourself time to adjust.

Cooking at home

Try cooking at home more often, such as making your own bread, pasta sauces, soups and cakes to facilitate a drastic reduction in your salt intake. Remember! Don't add salt at the table or during cooking. Sea salt and rock salt should also be avoided as these are just as high in salt. Avoid salty sauces such as soya sauce and tomato ketchup and use fresh, frozen or dried herbs, spices, chilli, garlic, pepper, vinegar, lemon or lime juice to add flavour instead.

⇨ The above information is reprinted with kind permission from Consensus Action on Salt and Health (CASH). Visit www.actiononsalt.org.uk for more.

© *Consensus Action on Salt and Health (CASH)*

CONSENSUS ACTION ON SALT AND HEALTH

Healthy hydration guide

Information from the British Nutrition Foundation.

Water is essential for life and it is very important to get the right amount of fluid to be healthy. However, there are lots of mixed messages about how much and what to drink, and this can be confusing. Do I really need to drink eight glasses of water on top of all my other drinks? Is it true that tea and coffee do not count towards my fluid intake? The answer to both these questions is no! The BNF 'healthy hydration guide' can help you choose a healthy balance of drinks.

This article also looks at why fluid is important, the effects of different drinks on health, and the needs of particular groups of people in the population. The information here is generally for healthy adults.

Why do you need water?

Your body is nearly two-thirds water and so it is really important that you consume enough fluid to stay hydrated and healthy. If you don't get enough fluid you may feel tired, get headaches and not perform at your best. 'Fluid' includes not only water from the tap or in a bottle, but also other drinks that give you water such as tea, coffee, milk, fruit juices and soft drinks. You also get water from the food you eat – on average food provides about 20% of your total fluid intake.

How much do you need?

The amount of fluid you need depends on many things, including the weather, how much physical activity you do and your age, but generally you should drink about 1.2 litres (six to eight glasses) of fluid per day (on top of the water provided by food you eat). You can get water from nearly all fluid that you drink, apart from stronger alcoholic drinks such as wine and spirits.

Can you drink too much?

Yes – drinking excessive amounts of fluid is not helpful and, in rare cases, can be dangerous. If you are passing urine frequently and your urine is very pale, you may be drinking more than you need.

Does it matter which drinks you choose?

When you choose your drinks it is important to be aware that although they all provide water and some also contain essential vitamins and minerals, they may also provide energy (calories). These calories contribute to your daily calorie intake in the same way as those from the foods you eat. It is also important to look after your teeth, and consuming sugar-containing drinks too often can potentially harm your teeth, especially if you don't brush teeth regularly with fluoride toothpaste. It is also important to be aware that some drinks are acidic (e.g. fruit juice and carbonated drinks) and that this may cause dental erosion (damage to tooth enamel) if they are consumed frequently. For children, the use of a straw lessens the contact with teeth.

Drinking water

Drinking water is a great choice because it delivers fluid without adding calories or potentially damaging teeth.

Tea and coffee

Drinking tea or coffee also delivers water, and even though these drinks can contain caffeine, in moderate amounts caffeine doesn't affect hydration. Pregnant women are advised to consume no more than 200mg of caffeine a day. This is equivalent to about two mugs of instant coffee or about two and a half mugs of tea. Other hot drinks such as herbal teas, hot chocolates and malted drinks can provide water. If these drinks are sweetened with sugar it increases their calorie content. The sugar also increases their potential to damage teeth if good dental hygiene is not practised.

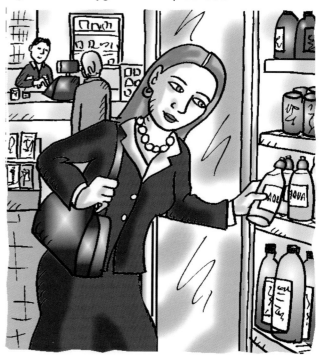

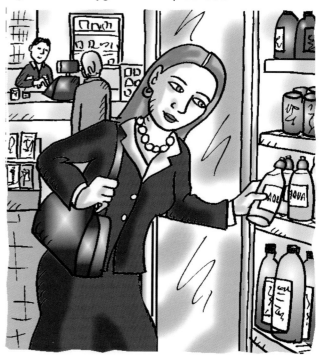

BRITISH NUTRITION FOUNDATION

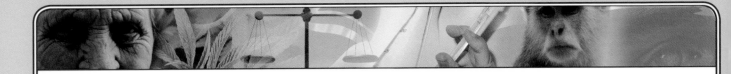

Milk

Milk contains lots of essential nutrients such as protein, B vitamins and calcium, as well as being a source of water. However, it can also contain saturated fat and so it's a good idea for adults and older children to choose semi-skimmed (less than 2% fat), 1% or skimmed milks. For children between the ages of one and two years, the recommended milk is whole milk. From two years onwards semi-skimmed milk can be introduced gradually. Skimmed and 1% milks are not suitable for children until they are at least five years old because they have less vitamin A and are lower in calories.

Fruit juices and smoothies

Fruit juices and smoothies give you water plus some vitamins, minerals and natural plant substances from the fruit. Smoothies may also contain pureed fruit, which adds fibre. These drinks can also count towards your five-a-day. One 150ml glass of fruit juice counts as one portion, and smoothies that contain at least 150ml of fruit juice and 80g crushed/pulped fruit count as two portions. Because fruit juices and smoothies contain sugar (and therefore calories) and can be acidic, they can potentially harm teeth.

Soft drinks

Soft drinks are a source of water but, if they contain sugar, this adds to your calorie intake and the sugar can potentially damage teeth if the drinks are consumed frequently. It's a good idea to limit consumption of standard sugar-containing soft drinks and to choose lower sugar or sugar-free (low-calorie) versions instead.

Alcoholic drinks

Alcoholic drinks contain water, but drinking alcohol increases the amount of water you lose as urine, so drinks with a high alcohol content, such as wines and spirits, are not the best choice to stay hydrated. Normal strength beers, lagers and ciders also cause an increased loss of water as urine. However, because they are more dilute, drinking them causes a net gain in water overall. It is still important to keep alcohol consumption within the recommended limits (no more than two to three units per day for women and no more than three to four units per day for men).

Food

Food – it may be a surprise to learn that we get on average 20% of our total water intake from food! Some foods have a high water content, especially fruits and vegetables, which are usually more than 80% water. Foods like soups and stews, which have lots of water added during preparation, are also a source of water.

So, food can provide extra water, on top of the six to eight glasses of fluid you should drink a day.

How can I tell if I am getting enough water?

Your body has special mechanisms to make sure you stay hydrated. Feeling thirsty is your body's way of telling you that you need to drink more. However, the easiest way to spot that you might not be getting enough water is if your urine is a dark yellow colour during the day. If you are getting enough water your urine should be a pale straw colour. So if it is darker than this or if you are urinating infrequently or passing very small amounts of urine, then you probably need to drink some more fluid. You also need to drink more if it is hot, or if your temperature is high due to physical activity or illness.

Do some people need more water than others?

Needs vary from one person to the next, but there are certain population groups who may need to pay particular attention to hydration.

Children

Children need plenty of fluid, despite their smaller body size, and they should be encouraged to drink regularly, especially if they are very active. Infants get their fluids from breast or formula milk, but will start to get some fluids from food when they move onto solids.

Older adults

Older adults may have a weaker sense of thirst and, if necessary, should be helped and encouraged to drink regularly.

Physical activity

Physical activity also increases the amount of fluid you need to consume in order to replace the water you lose as sweat. Water is fine for rehydrating after the kind of moderate exercise that most active people choose, and the majority of active people do not need special sports drinks to stay hydrated. However, for high-intensity exercise that lasts more than 40 minutes or so, drinks with a little added sugar and sodium (salt), such as sports drinks or home-made versions, may be better at replacing the extra fluid lost as sweat.

⇨ The above information is reprinted with kind permission from the British Nutrition Foundation. Visit www.nutrition.org.uk for more information on this and other related topics.

© British Nutrition Foundation

BRITISH NUTRITION FOUNDATION

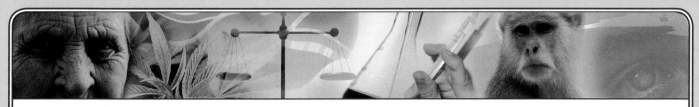

Food

Food lies at the centre of a very complex web that extends to every aspect of our existence, from the state of our countryside to the length of our lives.

With a growing population, climate change and the pressure we are putting on land, we will have to produce more food sustainably. We also need to provide the right information for people to make more informed choices about what they eat. Diet will have a huge impact not only on our health and our economy, but most importantly on sustainability.

To this end we will support and develop British farming and encourage sustainable food production, helping to enhance the competitiveness and resilience of the whole food chain, including farms and the fish industry, to ensure a secure, environmentally sustainable and healthy supply of food with improved standards of animal welfare.

We will need to work in partnership with a range of sectors from the food and farming industries, consumers, civil society and EU and international organisations.

Latest news

Supported by Defra, Eat Seasonably is all about inspiring and enabling people to eat more seasonal fruit and vegetables and helping them to grow their own. Visit the Eat Seasonably pages on Directgov to read more.

International context

As members of the EU, the UK food sector benefits from being part of the single market. It also means much of our food policy is influenced by EU legislation. As the biggest trading block in the world, the EU is a powerful figure on the international stage.

EU engagement therefore continues to be a priority, particularly in emphasising the importance of integrated food policy that meets the needs of Europe's citizens, and enables a competitive and sustainable food system that supports global food security.

The Department for International Development (DFID) and Defra work closely on influencing international action, and jointly sponsor a major international project led by Sir John Beddington, the UK's Chief Scientist, to address the question of how a global population of nine billion can all be fed healthily and sustainably. The Foresight project on Global Food and Farming Futures is due to report its findings in late 2010 or early 2011.

Challenges to the food system

⇨ The sector is heavily dependent on oil, energy and water, all increasingly scarce, and telecoms and transport where reliability and diversity of supply are essential.

⇨ Agriculture contributes to climate change: direct emissions from agriculture accounted for about 8% of UK greenhouse gas emissions in 2008.

⇨ Diet-related ill health costs the NHS an estimated £7 billion a year, with further costs to the wider economy through inability to work.

⇨ While consumers are increasingly interested in healthy eating, on current trends 40% of the UK population would be obese by 2025, and 60% by 2050.

⇨ 70,000 premature deaths a year could be avoided if, nationally, our diets matched nutritional guidelines on salt, fat, sugar and fruit and vegetable consumption.

⇨ Waste is a food chain issue – 8.3 million tonnes of food and drink is wasted by consumer each year, 5.3 million tonnes of this is avoidable.

⇨ With the global population estimated to increase from six billion to nine billion by 2050, the Food and Agriculture Organization (FAO) estimates global food production will have to increase by 70% compared to 2005–07 levels. Increasing availability of, and access to, existing food supplies, including by minimising waste along the food chain, will also be important. Already, over one billion people globally face hunger and undernourishment.

Economic significance of the food sector

⇨ The agri-food sector contributed £84.6 billion to the economy in 2008, 7.1% of the total and including the UK's largest manufacturing sector.

DEFRA

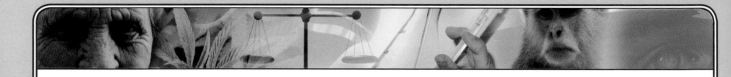

⇨ Three million people are employed in food and farming, of which 2.4 million are in the retail and food service sectors.

⇨ Consumer expenditure on food and drink was £177 billion in 2009.

⇨ The UK exported £13.2 billion worth of food and drink in 2008.

⇨ The UK imported £31.6 billion worth of food and drink in 2008.

26 October 2010

⇨ The above information is reprinted with kind permission from the Department for Environment, Food and Rural Affairs. Visit www.defra.gov.uk for more.

© Crown Copyright

Food and climate change

Sustain has taken a keen interest in the rapidly accumulating evidence about the contribution of food and farming to climate change.

Our food system is a very significant contributor to greenhouse gas emissions. The figures are startling.

⇨ The United Nations Food and Agriculture Organization (FAO) has calculated that, globally, agriculture generates 30% of total man-made emissions of greenhouse gases, including half of methane emissions and more than half of the emissions of nitrous oxide.

⇨ In the EU, over 30% of the greenhouse gases from consumer purchases come from the food and drink sector.

⇨ Latest conservative estimates from the Food Climate Research Network in the UK suggest that almost one-fifth of the UK's total greenhouse gas emissions are associated with our food and drink.

The emissions come not just from the transport of food, but from every stage of the chain – the conversion of land to agricultural use, the energy used to make fertilisers, pesticides and farm machinery, the impact of agriculture on the soil (a natural carbon store), food processing, transport, refrigeration, retail, domestic use of food and waste from all the different stages. These are complex problems with no single solution. A growing body of evidence, however, indicates that emissions from the food sector can be significantly reduced if we were all to shift towards eating the following:

Less meat and dairy, and more food from plants

Products from farmed animals – meat and dairy products such as milk and cheese – are among the most energy-intensive and greenhouse-gas intensive food products of all. According to the latest figures from the United Nations, animal farming globally causes more greenhouse gas emissions than all of the cars, lorries and planes in the world put together, and the impact is increasing. This is partly due to methane gas from the digestive systems of ruminants (cows and sheep burping), but also due to large areas of forest being cleared to grow grain and beans for livestock (including cows, pigs and chickens) to eat.

Local and seasonal food

Locally grown and prepared food can cut down on fuel use in 'food miles' and makes it easier to identify and support environmentally benign food production methods. Buying local produce also means that the food is less likely to be associated with the greenhouse gas caused by recent land conversion. Seasonal food need not be imported, does not require energy-intensive conditions such as heated greenhouses, can be produced organically, and reduces the likelihood of energy-intensive methods of storage and transport such as refrigeration and air-freighting.

In the EU, over 30% of the greenhouse gases from consumer purchases come from the food and drink sector

Food, such as organic, grown without artificial chemicals

Organic production methods are usually less energy-intensive than industrial agriculture. They do not use artificial fertiliser, which takes an enormous amount of energy and water to produce and results in emissions of the powerful greenhouse gas nitrous oxide.

10 March 2010

⇨ The above information is reprinted with kind permission from Sustain. Visit www.sustainweb.org for more information.

© Sustain

DEFRA / SUSTAIN

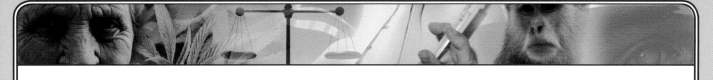

Food and drink: greener choices

Information from Directgov.

Food accounts for nearly a third of most people's effect on climate change. It also adds to many other environmental problems, like water pollution. You can help by reducing waste, choosing foods with a lower impact on climate change and opting for sustainable seafood.

Waste less food

The average UK family spends around £480 a year on food and drink that could have been used but is thrown away. Wasting food not only costs you money but also wastes the energy and resources needed to produce, package, store and transport it.

Cutting food waste benefits the environment. If everyone stopped wasting food that could be eaten, it would reduce CO_2 emissions as much as taking one in four cars off UK roads.

Visit the 'Love Food Hate Waste' website (www.lovefoodhatewaste.com) for recipes and practical tips to help you waste less food.

> **Wasted food and drink**
>
> £12 billion worth of food and drink that could have been used is thrown away every year.

Choose climate-friendly foods

The following tips can help you choose food with a lower carbon footprint:

⇨ Meat and dairy foods have a much bigger effect on climate change and the environment than most grains, pulses, fruit and vegetables.

⇨ Buying fresh and unprocessed foods can mean fewer carbon emissions, because processing food and freezing or refrigerating it uses a lot of energy.

⇨ Buying food grown outdoors in season can help reduce emissions, because it doesn't need heated greenhouses.

Transporting food

Food from a long way away doesn't necessarily have a big carbon footprint. Food transported long distances by boat (like bananas or apples), or food imported when it's in season abroad, can have a smaller footprint than:

⇨ food produced closer to home in heated greenhouses;

⇨ food that needs to be frozen or refrigerated, especially for long periods.

However, where food has been produced, stored and transported in similar ways, choosing food that hasn't travelled as far could help reduce CO_2 emissions.

Can healthy eating help the environment?

For many people, a diet with less saturated fat and more fruit and vegetables would be a healthy choice. This could also be a greener choice if you cut down on saturated fats by reducing the proportion of meat and dairy products you eat.

Buy sustainable fish

Worldwide, three-quarters of wild marine fisheries are fully or over-exploited. Estimates suggest that many of

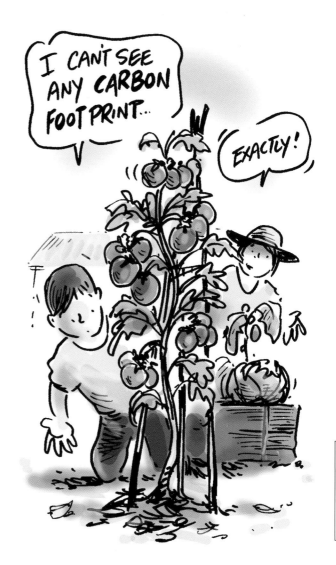

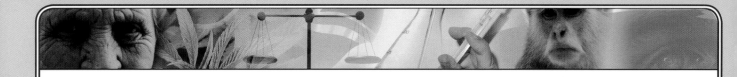

the world's commercial fisheries are likely to collapse in less than 50 years unless over-fishing is stopped.

You can help by buying seafood that has been sustainably produced. Find sustainable seafood in shops and restaurants by:

⇨ looking for labels that show seafood has been sustainably sourced, like the Marine Stewardship Council logo;

⇨ asking your retailer or restaurant owner if they have sustainable seafood options;

⇨ looking up recipes and advice on buying sustainable seafood at the Marine Stewardship Council website (www.msc.org).

Choose wildlife and environment-friendly food

Some food is made in ways that are more wildlife-friendly, for example without using pesticides. Other food supports the countryside and local communities, for example by creating local jobs. Find these by:

⇨ looking for labels like LEAF, organic and the Marine Stewardship Council;

⇨ choosing retailers that are trying to stock greener food.

If you can't find greener choices, you could ask your local shops to start stocking them. Showing an interest can encourage retailers to do more.

Buying from producers

Buying directly, for example at a farmers' market, means you can ask producers how their food is produced. Try looking for food:

⇨ from farmers who give high priority to looking after wildlife on their farm;

⇨ produced in a way which helps conserve rural landscapes, like upland sheep or cattle grazing.

Other ways of making greener food choices

Other things you can do include:

Cut down on car trips for food shopping

13 per cent of carbon emissions from transporting food come from individuals driving to the shops. Reducing shopping trips by car will help reduce carbon emissions, congestion and local air pollution.

Compost food waste

More than a third of household rubbish is kitchen or garden waste. Most of this ends up in landfill, where it gives off methane – a gas which has a big effect on climate change. However, when this waste is composted it doesn't give off methane.

Drink tap water

UK mains drinking water meets very high standards, uses around 300 times less energy than bottled water and doesn't leave bottles as waste.

Packaging can help preserve food – but it uses resources and can damage wildlife. 'Greener packaging choices' on the Directgov website has ideas on how you can reduce packaging waste.

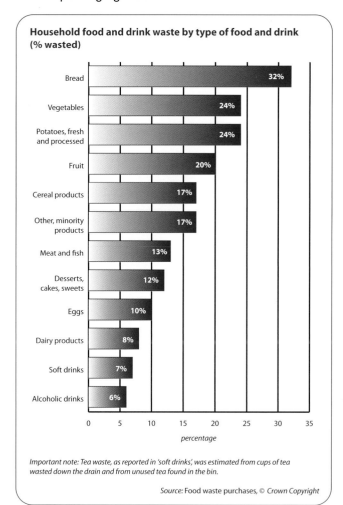

Household food and drink waste by type of food and drink (% wasted)

Type	Percentage
Bread	32%
Vegetables	24%
Potatoes, fresh and processed	24%
Fruit	20%
Cereal products	17%
Other, minority products	17%
Meat and fish	13%
Desserts, cakes, sweets	12%
Eggs	10%
Dairy products	8%
Soft drinks	7%
Alcoholic drinks	6%

percentage

Important note: Tea waste, as reported in 'soft drinks', was estimated from cups of tea wasted down the drain and from unused tea found in the bin.

Source: Food waste purchases, © Crown Copyright

Store and cook food efficiently

Defrosting your fridge regularly and putting lids on saucepans when cooking can save energy. 'Top tips on saving energy' on the Directgov website has more advice on ways you can save energy in the kitchen.

⇨ The above information is reprinted with kind permission from Directgov. Visit www.direct.gov.uk for more information.

DIRECTGOV

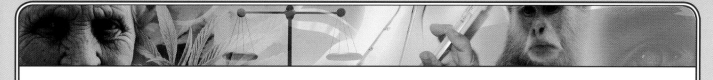

How do I know it's organic?

Information from the Soil Association.

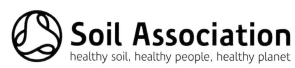

Soil Association
healthy soil, healthy people, healthy planet

'Organic' is a term defined by law. Any food products labelled as organic must meet a strict set of standards which define what farmers and food manufacturers can and cannot do in the production of organic food.

Organic products sold in the UK must by law display a certification symbol or number. Health and beauty and textile products are exempt from this law, so it is important to look for a genuine certification symbol for assurance that the product is truly organic.

Soil Association organic symbol

The Soil Association organic symbol can be found on 80% of UK organic food products. The Soil Association symbol tells you that produce has met and in some important areas exceeded minimum government requirements. Our standards cover every stage of production from the farm until it gets to your fork. They are continually developed to raise the quality of organic food.

UK certifier codes

Each certifier within the UK is given a UK code – the Soil Association is GB-ORG-05. The number awarded has nothing to do with stringency of standards. Legally, a company does not need to show a certification symbol on the pack but if the product has been produced and/ or processed in the UK they must show the UK code.

Imported products

There are many certification bodies throughout the world, active in certifying and promoting organic food. When one of our licensees wishes to use an ingredient either from another country or that has been certified by another body, we need to know that the product has been produced to the same or equivalent standards as the Soil Association's. We do this by either requesting information or directly inspecting the farm or company.

What information do you ask for?

Typically, we ask for the report written by the certification body after inspection to check all our relevant standards have been met. If our standards, or equivalent standards, have not been met then the product/ingredient cannot be used. The other option is to ask the existing certifier to confirm that our specific additional standard requirements have been met. We usually provide them with a document, which lists where our standards are

different and additional inspection requirements are necessary.

What checks do you make?

When deeming meat and dairy produce as equivalent, the major checks are:

⇨ Ensuring the animals have access to pasture.

⇨ Making sure organophosphate and organochlorine aren't used. On some farms (organic and non-organic) they are used to stop parasites like mites, lice and sheep scab. However, these chemicals have harmful health effects on animals, the environment and us.

⇨ Organic farmers use clean rotational grazing systems to reduce the build up of parasites, select hardier breeds with greater resistance to pests and parasites and take great care with fencing to prevent the spread of sheep scab. In cases where animals have pest problems despite a farmer's best efforts, a limited range of vet treatments (injections and 'pour ons') can be used, provided strict withdrawal periods are observed in order to ensure animals do not suffer.

⇨ Ensuring our slaughter standards are met. These include: not allowing any tenderising substances prior to slaughter and ensuring all animals are stunned before slaughter. This process must cause unconsciousness and insensibility instantaneously, without distress, and until the animal dies.

About the Soil Association

The Soil Association was founded in 1946 by a group of farmers, scientists and nutritionists who observed a direct connection between the health of the soil, food, people and the environment. Today the Soil Association is the UK's leading organic organisation, with over 200 staff based in Bristol and Edinburgh. It is an educational charity with some 27,000 members, and its certification subsidiary, Soil Association Certification Ltd, certifies over 80% of organic farming and food processing in the UK.

⇨ The above information is reprinted with kind permission from the Soil Association. Visit www. soilassociation.org for more information.

© *Soil Association*

THE SOIL ASSOCIATION

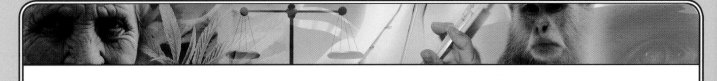

The great organic con trick

Organic produce is better for you? Robert Johnston explodes five myths about its benefits.

Interest groups claim that organic food is healthier and better for the environment, but many of such claims are myths.

Myth: Organic food is healthier

Actually, scientific studies show more health risks from organic food than conventional food. This month in California, for instance, Salmonella was found in organic fertilisers which could contaminate fruit and vegetables.

In 2003, Dutch scientists established that organic chickens and conventional birds had the same rate of infection with Salmonella even though many organic farmers vaccinate their chickens against the bug. In 2006, other Dutch scientists found that as many as three-quarters of organic chickens were infected with parasites.

Organic manure can also carry the dangerous bacteria Campylobacter, which causes stomach infections, vomiting and diarrhoea. The Danish National Veterinary Laboratory found Campylobacter in 100 per cent of organic chicken flocks but only 36.7 per cent of conventional chicken flocks.

Organic and free-range poultry are more likely to be exposed to bird-flu, so the Government now allows organic chickens to be kept indoors.

Myth: Organic farming is good for the environment

In Britain, the yield of wheat from organic farms is only half that from conventional farms. If all our food was organic, we would have to grub up hedgerows and cut down forests just to produce enough food. We would use twice the water, do at least twice the ploughing and use twice the amount of petrol and diesel.

Two organically raised cows burp the same amount of methane as three conventionally fed cows and methane is 20 times more powerful as a greenhouse gas than CO_2.

Most modern pesticides are biodegradable, but 'natural' pesticides, like copper, stay in the soil forever.

Myth: Organic farmers don't use pesticides

The Canadian Food Safety Agency found pesticide residues in as many organic baby foods as conventional baby food and the highest pesticide level was in an organic food.

Organic farmers spray crops with 'natural' pesticides such as the noxious microbe BT, which kills bees, ladybirds and butterflies as well as pests by releasing the same toxin made by genetically modified plants. If inhaled, it can cause bronchitis and worsen asthma.

Organic farmers treat fungus with copper solutions which also poison earthworms and friendly bacteria. They also use Derris which can cause Parkinson's disease; pyrethroids, which cause tumours in mice; and potassium permanganate which kills fish.

Myth: Organic food does not contain additives

At least three dozen 'E' numbers are allowed as additives, preservatives, flavourings, binders, anti-caking agents, antioxidants and processing agents in 'organic' food.

For cleaning and disinfection, organic farmers use the same substances as conventional farmers, including formaldehyde, caustic soda, nitric and phosphoric acid, quicklime, alcohol and other highly toxic chemicals that can contaminate food.

Organically reared animals can have up to a quarter of their daily food from non-organic sources and all organic food can contain five per cent of conventional ingredients.

Myth: The demand for organic food is at an all-time high

Even with the support of TV chefs Jamie Oliver and Hugh Fearnley-Wittingstall, only two per cent of the food sold in Britain is organic. At the end of the Second World War all our food was organic so, in fact, demand has actually gone down by 98 per cent over the last 60 years.

Despite the vocal campaigns by celebrity chefs, only about one per cent of the chickens sold in Britain are organic. Nor does buying organic food support British farmers since 70 per cent of it is imported.

Organic food is a fashion and lifestyle choice. It is probably no worse for you or the environment than conventional foods, but organic proponents should get their facts straight and stop using dubious claims about 'natural' meaning 'better' and stick to the facts.

⇨ The above information is reprinted with kind permission from The First Post. Visit www.thefirstpost.co.uk for more information.

© The First Post

THE FIRST POST

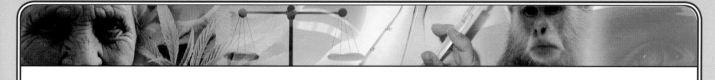

The great organic myths rebutted

Rob Johnston argued that organic foods are not as good as supporters claim. His article sparked heated debate. Now Peter Melchett of the Soil Association puts the case for their defence.

Fact one: Organic farming is good for the environment

Organic farming is not perfect; it was only developed 60 years ago, and we still have much to learn. Over those years, organic research has been starved of funding because most investment went first into developing pesticides and then into GM crops. Organic farming was started by scientists and farmers who wanted to develop what we would now call a more sustainable way of producing food. Their main concern was with the link between healthy soils, healthy food and human health. However, those pioneers did create a farming system that has clear environmental benefits. Organic farming is better for wildlife on farms. The science is clear cut. Scientific literature reviews have found that, overall, organic farms have 30 per cent more wild species, and 50 per cent higher numbers of those species. Based on scientific research, the Government says that organic farming has clear environmental benefits – better for wildlife, lower pollution from sprays, produces fewer dangerous wastes and less carbon dioxide. The Sustainable Development Commission says that organic certification represents 'the gold standard' for sustainable food production. I farmed non-organically for more than 30 years, and switched to organic, mainly to try to bring back wildlife on the farm. We have far more birds, and data on hares before and after switching to organic show numbers doubled from 20 to 40. This year we found 56.

Fact two: Organic farming is more sustainable

Last week's article contained several errors – for example, the statement that organic tomatoes take double the amount of energy to produce is wrong, as were the figures for different types of tomato. The information on the climate change impact of organic food omitted one of the key benefits of organic farming: storing carbon in the soil. When this is included, the climate change impact of organic food goes down by between 12 and 80 per cent. Government-funded studies have shown that across a range of sectors, organic farming uses 26 per cent less energy than non-organic farming to produce the same amount of food, and the Government agrees that organic farming is better for climate change. The article ignored the extraordinary challenges we face. We must drastically reduce greenhouse gas emissions from the farming and food industries – by 80 per cent by 2050. We have to adapt to a world with declining oil and gas supplies. We have to help mitigate the effects of climate change, for example by reducing flooding and cutting demand for fresh water. We have to adapt to a world of more extreme and unpredictable weather. How we do this is the challenge.

Fact three: Organic farming doesn't use pesticides

We've never claimed this! The Soil Association's rules allow farmers to use four pesticides, with permission. Non-organic farming uses more than 300. The vast majority of organic farmers have no need for sprays. If all farming was organic, spraying would fall by 98 per cent. Organic sprays are mainly used on potatoes and in orchards. Those we allow are either of natural origin (rotenone and soft soap) or simple chemical products – copper compounds and sulphur. The active ingredients in rotenone and soft soap break down rapidly when exposed to sunlight, minimising risk to the environment. Copper and sulphur occur naturally in the soil, and most copper is applied by non-organic farmers to correct copper deficiencies. None is found in organic food.

Despite the wet weather and greatly increased risk of disease last year, only three per cent of Soil Association farmers and two per cent of organic crops were sprayed. Our goal is to use no sprays at all.

Fact four: Pesticide levels in conventional food are dangerous

I'd say certainly risky, and potentially dangerous. In the EU, one food item in 30 contains levels above European legal limits. Nearly 40 pesticides, which we were promised were safe, have been banned or withdrawn from use over the past decade. People who want to reduce their exposure to potentially harmful pesticides can buy organic food. A US study showed that within one day of switching to an organic diet no traces of pesticides could be found in children's urine. When the children switched back to a non-organic diet, pesticides were found immediately.

Cocktails of sprays are not tested when pesticides are passed as 'safe', and research has confirmed they pose a risk. Average male fertility has fallen by 50 per cent, coinciding with the use of pesticides. There are alternative views – a government adviser blamed 'too much time riding bikes, sitting down too much

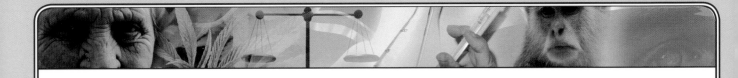

and wearing tight underpants'. Science cannot prove there is no risk from pesticides. In the absence of clear scientific evidence either way, people who think that the accepted nutritional differences or absence of pesticides and artificial additives in organic food will benefit them or their children, should buy organic.

Fact five: Organic farming is healthier

In terms of food safety, the Food Standards Agency says there is no difference between organic and non-organic food. The animal welfare organisation Compassion in World Farming says: 'Organic farming has the potential to offer the very highest standards of animal welfare.' It believes that the Soil Association's welfare standards are 'leaders in the field'. Because animals are kept in better conditions, always free range, there is no need for the routine use of antibiotics, and such use is banned. The World Health Organization says that: 'There is growing concern that antibiotic residues in meat and dairy products could result in antibiotic resistance in bacteria prevalent in humans, reducing the effectiveness of antibiotics used to treat human disease.' The most bizarre claim in last week's piece was that 'Disease is the major reason why organic animals are half the weight of conventionally reared animals – so organic farming is not necessarily a boon to animal welfare'. There is no truth in this. An organic steak or chicken are the same size as non-organic – have a look in the shops! Organic animals suffer no more disease, and frequently less, than non-organic.

Fact six: Organic food contains more nutrients

Published research shows that, on average, organic food contains higher levels of vitamin C and essential minerals such as calcium, magnesium, iron and chromium, as well as cancer-fighting antioxidants. Organic milk is naturally higher in Omega 3 fatty acids, Vitamin E, Vitamin A (beta-carotene) and some other antioxidants than non-organic milk.

Diseases such as eczema, asthma and allergies are affecting more and more children. Ten per cent of children in the EU now suffer from eczema. Following research in Sweden, a Dutch government-funded study published last November showed a 36 per cent lower incidence of eczema in children fed on organic dairy products compared with children consuming non-organic dairy products.

Organic standards prohibit a host of additives that researchers say may be harmful to our health, such as hydrogenated fat, monosodium glutamate and artificial flavourings and colourings. Recent Food Standards Agency-funded research found that some common additives can cause hyperactivity in children. You can avoid a wide range and large quantity of potentially allergenic or harmful additives if you eat organic food.

Fact seven: The demand for organic food is growing

Organic is still small. But local and direct organic sales are growing at 32 per cent per annum. In 2006 (the latest figures available), retail and catering sales were worth £1,937m – on average the retail market has grown 27 per cent per year over the past decade, and over the past few years, the proportion of the market supplied by UK farmers has grown. This is no longer simply a middle-class market. Over 50 per cent of people in lower-income groups are buying organic food, and if they buy direct from farmers via box schemes or farm shops, it need not be more expensive than the same non-organic food in supermarkets. Three-quarters of parents buy organic baby food, which makes up about half the total sold. Many parents and school governors have opted for at least part of school dinners being sourced from organic farms.

Organic farming is helping to reverse the decline in the UK's agricultural workforce, which has fallen by 80 per cent over the past 50 years. Organic farms in the UK provide on average more than 30 per cent more jobs per farm than equivalent non-organic farms – organic farmers tend to be younger, more optimistic and include more women. The choice we face is between oil-based farming with nitrogen fertiliser, or solar-powered organic systems. Producing one ton of nitrogen releases the equivalent of 6.7 tons of CO_2. The raw material used to produce nitrogen fertiliser is, currently, increasingly scarce natural gas. UK farming uses three million tons of nitrogen fertiliser annually, half of which is imported. Organic farming is based on renewable processes on the farm, using clover to fix nitrogen and to build soil organic matter.

Recent research suggests that if all farming was organic, the slight decrease in yields in the northern hemisphere would be more than matched by overall increases elsewhere, leading to a slight increase in total food production. Long-term trials in the US found organic yields matching those from non-organic systems, with organic farming outperforming non-organic in drought years. Even with the uncertainties, in a world of increasing scarcity of fossil fuels, organic farming provides the only environmentally, or economically, sustainable system of feeding the world. Organic farming and food do not have all the answers. But solar-powered, animal and wildlife friendly, pesticide- and additive-free farming and food, is where we're heading.

8 May 2008

© *The Independent*

THE INDEPENDENT

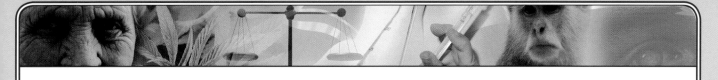

Going vegetarian

There's more to being a vegetarian than giving up meat. Like everyone else, vegetarians need to ensure they eat a balanced and varied diet.

Studies have shown that, on average, vegetarians have a lower risk of obesity, heart disease, high blood pressure and diabetes than meat eaters.

Around 5% of the UK population is vegetarian, with the highest proportion being teenage girls.

Vegetarians live on a diet of grains, pulses, nuts, seeds, fruit and vegetables, dairy products and eggs.

They don't eat any meat, poultry, game, fish, shellfish or crustacea (such as crab or lobster), or animal by-products (such as gelatine).

There are three main types of vegetarian:

⇨ Lacto-ovo-vegetarians eat both dairy products and eggs. This is the most common type of vegetarian diet.

⇨ Lacto-vegetarians eat dairy products but not eggs.

⇨ Vegans do not eat dairy products, eggs, or any other animal product.

Pulses

Peas, beans and lentils are known as pulses. They contain fibre, protein and carbohydrate and are low in fat. They are also a good source of B vitamins.

Healthy lifestyle

'Many vegetarians, as long as they eat a balanced diet, are as healthy as, if not healthier than, the general population,' says registered dietitian Ursula Arens, a spokesperson for the British Dietetic Association.

A vegetarian diet is suitable for everyone regardless of their age, although dietitians do not recommend an entirely vegan diet for infants and young children.

All children between six months and five years, regardless of their diet, are recommended to take vitamin drops containing vitamins A, C and D. You can buy these at any pharmacy.

'There is a concern that children on a strict vegan diet may not get all the nutrients they need. This means they can be underweight and grow more slowly, or have stunted growth,' says Arens.

It's also important to take extra care during pregnancy and breastfeeding to make sure you and your baby are getting enough vitamin D and B12.

Getting started

While there's no harm in switching to a vegetarian diet overnight, you may prefer to do it gradually. Some people give up red meat first, then poultry, then fish.

Others eat vegetarian food one day a week at first, then two or three days, and eventually every day. Do it in a way that suits you.

Get a vegetarian cookbook or look up recipes online. Whether you need simple step-by-step instructions or can follow more complex recipes, there are enough options for a vegetarian diet to give you plenty of variety.

Being a vegetarian is also a way of life and an opportunity to take a fresh look at food. Visit your local supermarket and health-food shop and get to know as many different vegetarian foods as possible, including meat alternatives.

If you've grown up eating meat, you'll have to change some of your habits. The easiest way to stay healthy is to learn what your body needs.

To avoid any embarrassment when friends are cooking for you, remember to let them know in advance that you are a vegetarian.

Good sources of protein

⇨ Soya-based foods, such as tofu and soya milk.

⇨ Beans, lentils and chickpeas.

⇨ Seeds, nuts, nut butters and nut milk.

⇨ Eggs.

⇨ Meat replacement products, such as Quorn.

A variety of protein from different sources is necessary to get the right mixture of amino acids, which are used to build and repair the body's cells.

Healthy eating

The main healthy eating guidelines for vegetarians are the same as for everybody else.

A healthy diet includes plenty of fruit, vegetables and grains such as wheat and rice (preferably wholegrain), moderate amounts of foods containing protein and dairy products, and only a small amount of foods containing fat and sugar.

The Food Standards Agency's eatwell plate (see page 2) shows you how much to eat from each major food group.

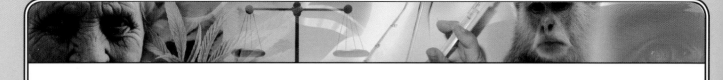

Common nutritional deficiencies in vegetarian and vegan diets include vitamin D, vitamin B12 and iron.

Vitamin D is generated by sunlight on our skin. If you don't go outside much or if you have dark skin, you should include fortified margarine or spreads and fortified breakfast cereals in your diet and take vitamin D supplements.

Vitamin B12, which helps the body grow and repair itself, is mainly found in meat, fish and dairy products. To get enough vitamin B12, try to eat fortified breakfast cereal, soya foods or yeast extract regularly.

Most vegetarians do not need to take food supplements as long as they eat a balanced diet. But getting the balance right can be more difficult for vegans, says Arens. 'Because they don't eat dairy products, vegans need to plan their diet carefully to ensure they get enough vitamin B12.'

If you eat the right foods in the right proportions with plenty of variety, you shouldn't have any problems achieving a healthy, balanced diet.

14 October 2009

⇨ Reproduced by kind permission of the Department of Health.

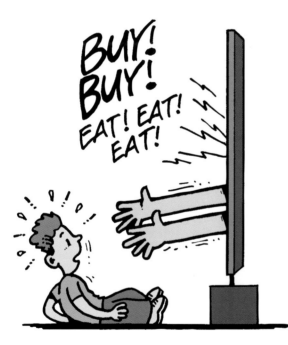

Watershed ban on junk food advertising would help tackle childhood obesity

Information from the British Heart Foundation.

Children see 37 per cent less junk food advertising on TV compared with five years ago, according to an Ofcom report. But the BHF say a complete watershed ban is needed to deal effectively with rising childhood obesity.

Ofcom's review shows that advertising bans during children's programmes and on dedicated children's channels are working to prevent children being influenced by junk food firms.

But it also shows that just over half of children's viewing time is during adult airtime and that the impact of the ban on older children, aged ten to 15, is much less.

BHF chief executive Peter Hollins said: 'Banning junk food adverts during children's programmes has clearly had some positive effect. But the Government can – and should – go further.

Children see 37 per cent less junk food advertising on TV compared with five years ago, according to an Ofcom report

'The report showed the ban was less effective for older children, who watch TV shows like *The X Factor* and *Britain's Got Talent* where restrictions don't apply. Yet these children are just starting to make their own choices about what they eat and are beginning to buy their own snacks and meals.

'A complete ban on junk food advertising before 9pm would better protect them from the influence of slick advertising campaigns while they learn how to choose between treats and foods that are good for them.'

26 July 2010

⇨ The above information is reprinted with kind permission from the British Heart Foundation. Visit www.bhf.org.uk for more information.

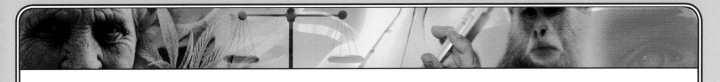

Mums hoodwinked by manipulative food manufacturers

Nine out of ten (92%) mums are misled by tactics manufacturers use to market children's foods loaded with fat, salt and sugar, a British Heart Foundation survey revealed today.

The survey asked parents what they thought about statements such as 'free from artificial colours and preservatives' and 'a source of calcium, iron and six vitamins'.

It illustrates how the nation's mums believe they indicate a product is likely to be healthy. Yet the shocking truth behind such lines is:

⇨ Wholegrain – 76% of mums believe that 'wholegrain' means the product is likely to be healthy. For example Nestlé state that Honey Shreddies are 'wholegrain' and can 'keep your heart healthy and maintain a healthy body' yet a 45g average size serving contains more sugar (13.6g) than a ring doughnut (9.2g).

⇨ Source of calcium, iron and six vitamins – 63% of mums think this indicates the product is likely to be healthy. For example, Coco Pops use this line on their cereal and milk bars, yet per 100g they are higher in saturated fat and sugar than the average chocolate cake.

Nestlé state that Honey Shreddies are 'wholegrain' and can 'keep your heart healthy and maintain a healthy body' yet a 45g average size serving contains more sugar (13.6g) than a ring doughnut (9.2g)

⇨ No artificial flavourings, no artificial colourings – Nearly three in five (59%) mums believe this indicates the product is likely to be healthy. The Natural Confectionery Company packaging states that Jelly Snakes sweets have 'no artificial flavourings, no artificial colourings' and are 'natural'. Yet they contain more calories gram for gram than black treacle.

As part of its Food4Thought campaign the BHF examines how food manufacturers manipulate parents through distracting health-like claims to market breakfast foods and lunchbox snacks.

Peter Hollins, Chief Executive of the BHF, said: 'Mums are having the wool pulled over their eyes by food manufacturers.

'Smoke and mirror tactics means that foods targeted at children and high in fat, salt and sugar are being disguised with partial health claims suggesting they're a healthy choice. Regularly eating these types of foods could have serious implications for kids' future health.'

The survey also revealed that eight out of ten (84%) parents supported calls for a single, front-of-pack food labelling scheme.

'It's time for food companies to stop making excuses'

An independent review commissioned by the Food Standards Agency concluded that a single front-of-pack scheme combining traffic light colours, guideline daily amounts and the words high, medium and low would be the most helpful to shoppers. But many food companies are resisting this system of food labelling.

Peter Hollins said: 'Partial health claims and the mish mash of food labelling systems serve only to confuse shoppers about the nutritional value of what they're putting in their shopping baskets.

'It's time for food companies to stop making excuses, support one system and ensure shoppers are given "at a glance" information about the foods they're giving their kids.'

Natalie Rogers, aged 33 and a mum of two from Stratford-upon-Avon, said: 'When I go to the supermarket I'm faced with a barrage of different food labels and it's difficult to tell how bad a product is for my kids.

'If food companies truly cared about us as customers they would welcome a clear and consistent food labelling system which would help me make healthy food choices. Surely food companies have nothing to fear in clearly revealing what's in their products?'

20 December 2009

⇨ The above information is reprinted with kind permission from the British Heart Foundation. Visit www.bhf.org.uk for more information.

© British Heart Foundation

BRITISH HEART FOUNDATION

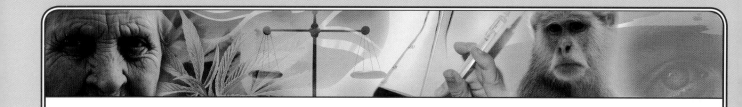

KEY FACTS

⇨ The UK population is eating less saturated fat, less trans-fat and less added sugar than it was ten years ago. (page 1)

⇨ When it comes to a healthy diet, balance is the key to getting it right. This means eating a wide variety of foods in the right proportions. (page 2)

⇨ Fats and sugar are both good sources of energy for the body. But when we eat too much of them we consume more energy than we burn, and this can mean that we put on weight. (page 3)

⇨ Eating at least five portions of fruit and vegetables a day can reduce the risk of heart disease, stroke and some cancers by up to 20%. (page 4)

⇨ Almost a third of children regularly go without breakfast before school and are more likely than classmates to be inactive, unfit and obese, research shows. (page 8)

⇨ There are EU-wide regulations that list the additives which have been tested and shown to be safe for use in food. (page 15)

⇨ According to recent research, more than two-fifths (43%) of shoppers say they eat five portions of fruit or vegetables a day as part of a healthy lifestyle. (page 17)

⇨ Children who have at least one obese parent are three to four times more likely to be obese themselves. (page 19)

⇨ One in every two people is now overweight or obese in almost half of OECD countries. Rates are projected to increase further and in some countries two out of three people will be obese within ten years. (page 21)

⇨ Many diets, especially crash diets, involve dramatically reducing the number of calories consumed. You may lose weight quickly but you risk losing muscle rather than fat. (page 22)

⇨ Adults should do at least 30 minutes of activity five times a week for general health benefits. To lose weight and keep it off, you need to do at least 60 minutes of activity regularly. (page 23)

⇨ The average man should eat no more than 30g of saturated fat a day and the average woman, no more than 20g. (page 24)

⇨ Adults need less than one gram of salt per day and children need even less, but most adults now eat between seven to ten grams per day, far more than needed. (page 25)

⇨ Your body is nearly two-thirds water and so it is really important that you consume enough fluid to stay hydrated and healthy. (page 27)

⇨ The agri-food sector contributed £84.6 billion to the economy in 2008, 7.1% of the total and including the UK's largest manufacturing sector. (page 29)

⇨ In the EU, over 30% of the greenhouse gases from consumer purchases come from the food and drink sector. (page 30)

⇨ The average UK family spends around £480 a year on food and drink that could have been used but is thrown away. Wasting food not only costs you money but also wastes the energy and resources needed to produce, package, store and transport it. (page 31)

⇨ UK mains drinking water meets very high standards, uses around 300 times less energy than bottled water and doesn't leave bottles as waste. (page 32)

⇨ Any food products labelled as organic must meet a strict set of standards which define what farmers and food manufacturers can and cannot do in the production of organic food. (page 33)

⇨ Around 5% of the UK population is vegetarian, with the highest proportion being teenage girls. (page 37)

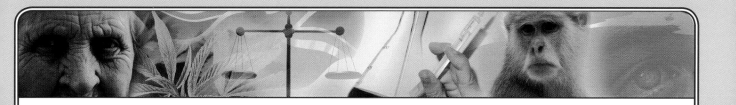

Additives

Additives are ingredients used in the preparation of processed foods. Some of these are extracted from naturally occurring materials, others are manufactured chemicals. They may be added to food to stop it going bad (preservatives), improve its appearance (for example by changing its colour) or to enhance its flavour. Other types of additives include thickeners, sweeteners, emulsifiers and anti-caking agents, and there are many more.

Body Mass Index (BMI)

An individual's body mass index is calculated by applying a formula to their weight and height to determine if they are within a healthy weight range. A healthy individual has a BMI of between 20 and 25. Someone with a BMI of 30 or above would be classed as obese.

Diet

The variety of food and drink that someone eats on a regular basis. The phrase 'on a diet' is also often used to refer to a period of controlling what one eats while trying to lose weight.

Fibre

Dietary fibre (sometimes called 'roughage') is the part of fruit, vegetables and wholefoods which cannot be digested by the body. It aids digestion by giving the gut bulk to squeeze against in order to move food through the digestive system. There are two types of fibre: soluble and insoluble.

Food poisoning

A range of illnesses, usually involving vomiting and diarrhoea symptoms, caused by ingesting bacteria though food and drink.

Junk food

'Junk' food is a widely-used term for unhealthy and fatty food with little nutritional value. It is usually associated with 'fast' or takeaway food.

Nutrition

The provision of materials needed by the body for growth, maintenance and sustaining life. Commonly when people talk about nutrition, they are referring to the healthy and balanced diet we all need to eat in order for the body to function properly.

Obesity

When someone is overweight to the extent that their BMI is 30 or above, they are classed as obese. Obesity is increasing in the UK and is associated with a number of health problems, including heart disease and diabetes.

Organic produce

Food that has been produced without the use of chemical fertilisers or pesticides. It takes many years for soil to become truly organic and free from any man-made chemicals. Organic food must meet certain legal standards before it can legitimately be called 'organic'.

Protein

Proteins are chains of amino acids that allow the body to build and repair body tissue. Protein is found in dairy foods, meat, fish and soya beans.

Starch

Starch is a complex carbohydrate found in potatoes, rice, corn, wheat and other foods. It is made up of glucose and allows animals and plants to store energy as fat.

Traffic light labelling

A new food labelling system, implemented by large food manufacturers and supermarkets to provide clear nutritional information to their consumers. Red, amber and green labels are used on food packaging to indicate how healthy that food is considered, with a green label indicating a very healthy food and red indicating a food that is high in salt, sugar or fats and which should therefore be enjoyed only in moderation.

Vegetarian

Someone who chooses not to eat any meat or meat-industry by-products (such as gelatine) for reasons of ethics, personal taste, health or a combination of these issues. A vegan does not eat any animal products at all, including meat and its by-products, eggs, honey and dairy.

Vitamins

Organic compounds that are essential to the body, but only in very small quantities. Most of the vitamins and minerals we need are provided through a balanced diet: however, some people choose to take additional vitamin supplements.

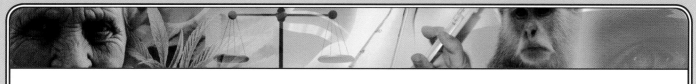

ACKNOWLEDGEMENTS

The publisher is grateful for permission to reproduce the following material.

While every care has been taken to trace and acknowledge copyright, the publisher tenders its apology for any accidental infringement or where copyright has proved untraceable. The publisher would be pleased to come to a suitable arrangement in any such case with the rightful owner.

Chapter One: Diet and Health

The nation's diet, © Crown copyright is reproduced with the permission of Her Majesty's Stationery Office, *A balanced diet,* © Crown copyright is reproduced with the permission of Her Majesty's Stationery Office – nhs. uk, *Diet and nutrition,* © PharmacyHealthLink, *Food poisoning,* © Food Ethics Council, *Food in schools,* © Crown copyright is reproduced with the permission of Her Majesty's Stationery Office, *32% of pupils skip breakfast before school, study finds,* © Guardian News and Media Limited 2010, *Breakfast,* © Crown copyright is reproduced with the permission of Her Majesty's Stationery Office, *Junk food fills children's lunchboxes,* © Guardian News and Media Limited 2010, *Buy healthier food,* © Crown copyright is reproduced with the permission of Her Majesty's Stationery Office – nhs.uk, *Food standards – labelling and composition,* © Crown copyright is reproduced with the permission of Her Majesty's Stationery Office, *Food additives,* © Sense about Science, *Healthy eating habits uncovered,* © Institute of Grocery Distribution, *Top doctor calls for urgent action on salt and fats in food,* © Guardian News and Media Limited 2010, *Obesity and the economics of prevention: fit not fat,* © Organisation for Economic Co-Operation and Development, *The truth about fad diets,* © Crown copyright is reproduced with permission of Her Majesty's Stationery Office – nhs.uk, *Saturated fat,* © British Nutrition Foundation, *Salt and your health,* © Consensus Action on Salt and Health (CASH), *Healthy hydration guide,* © British Nutrition Foundation.

Chapter Two: Ethical Eating

Food, © Crown copyright is reproduced with the permission of Her Majesty's Stationery Office, *Food and climate change,* © Sustain, *Food and drink: greener choices,* © Crown copyright is reproduced with the permission of Her Majesty's Stationery Office, *How do I know it's organic?,* © Soil Association, *The great organic con trick,* © The First Post, *The great organic myths rebutted,* © The Independent, *Going vegetarian,* © Crown copyright is reproduced with the permission of Her Majesty's Stationery Office – nhs.uk, *Watershed ban on junk food advertising would help tackle childhood obesity,* © British Heart Foundation, *Mums hoodwinked by manipulative food manufacturers,* © British Heart Foundation.

Illustrations

Pages 1, 21, 31: Simon Kneebone; pages 3, 27: Bev Aisbett; pages 4, 22, 38: Don Hatcher; pages 6, 14, 25: Angelo Madrid.

Cover photography

Left: © Jason Antony. Centre: © Carolina Farion. Right: © Zsuzsanna Kilian.

Additional acknowledgements

Research by Shivonne Gates.

Additional editorial by Carolyn Kirby on behalf of Independence.

And with thanks to the Independence team: Mary Chapman, Sandra Dennis and Jan Sunderland.

Lisa Firth
Cambridge
January, 2011

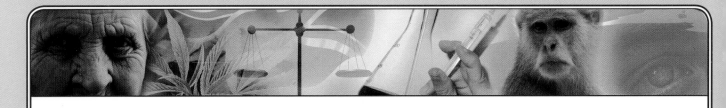

The following tasks aim to help you think through the issues surrounding diet and nutrition and provide a better understanding of the topic.

1 Read *A balanced diet* on pages 2–3 and look at the accompanying diagram. The eatwell plate is one tool used to encourage people to eat healthily. Devise another way of educating people about the different food groups which could be used to promote healthy eating. It could be a poster, a short rhyme or even a song – anything that could be used as part of a healthy eating campaign.

2 Imagine it is your responsibility to cook for a household containing two adults and two young children. One of the adults is a vegetarian. One of the children is a fussy eater and dislikes vegetables. Create a meal plan for the week, ensuring each member of the household is eating a balanced diet which they will enjoy (use the eatwell plate as a guide). When you have finished, compare your meals with a partner and discuss how easy or difficult you found it to come up with ideas.

3 Read *32% of pupils skip breakfast, study finds* and *Breakfast* on pages 8–9, then carry out a survey of the students in your year group to find out who eats breakfast before school. Ask respondents if they always have their breakfast, if they only have it sometimes or if they never have it. You could also ask what they would normally have for breakfast. Create a set of graphs to display your findings.

4 In recent years, the nutritional value of school dinners has come under scrutiny. Carry out your own research into the issue of school meals, looking at campaigns such as Jamie Oliver's 'Feed Me Better' project. How healthy are the meals served in your own school canteen? Do you think they could be improved?

5 Find out about Paul McCartney's Meat Free Monday campaign. How does it aim to help the environment? Take part in a Meat Free Monday and write about whether you found it easy or difficult to give up meat for a day.

6 Look at the eating habits of different countries around the world. Which countries have problems with the population's diet, obesity levels and nutrition-related health? Are there any cultural factors at play which might contribute to these problems? Have the governments of these countries taken any measures to change the nation's eating habits?

7 Create an information booklet warning people about the dangers of so-called 'fad' diets. You can use the information in *The truth about fad diets* on pages 22–23 to help you. Think about the reasons people choose to go on fad diets and how you might convince them that there are healthier ways of losing weight. Which healthy GP-recommended diet plans might they choose to follow instead? You could do some research into popular fad diets and include a summary of why each one is unhealthy and/or unsuccessful.

8 What is Body Mass Index (BMI) and how is it used to measure whether someone is a healthy weight? Is it a useful tool? Can you think of any problems with the way BMI is calculated?

9 'This house believes it is not the responsibility of the "nanny state" Government or the supermarkets to promote healthy eating – the consumer chooses which foods they buy and eat, and it is up to them to regulate their diet.' Debate this statement in two groups, with one group arguing in favour of the proposal and the other against it.

10 What are calories and where would you look for information about them on food you had purchased? How do people who want to lose weight use these to limit the amount they eat? Is calorie counting a useful way to lose weight?

11 Look at a TV guide. How many cookery and food-related programmes are shown on television in the course of a week? Do any cover healthy eating? Why do you think these programmes are so popular – do you think as a nation we have become obsessed with what we eat?

12 With a partner, role-play a radio interview on the topic of 'greener food'. The interviewee, a campaigner for an environmental charity, should give advice on how our food affects the environment, how we can purchase climate-friendly and sustainable food and how we can produce less waste.

13 Read *Going vegetarian* on page 37. How can vegetarians ensure they are getting all required nutrients in their diet? Create a booklet for new vegetarians, providing information on how to eat a balanced meat-free diet for good health. You might even choose to include some recipe suggestions! The Vegetarian Society's website (www.vegsoc.org) will have more information about nutrition for vegetarians.